Responsible Research

A GUIDE FOR COORDINATORS

Also available from Remedica:
Clinical Trials: A Practical Guide to Design, Analysis, and Reporting
The Clinical Research Survival Guide
Handbook of Clinical Trials

Published by Remedica
Commonwealth House, 1 New Oxford Street, London, WC1A 1NU, UK
Civic Opera Building, 20 North Wacker Drive, Suite 1642, Chicago, IL 60606, USA

info@remedicabooks.com
www.remedicabooks.com
Tel: +44 20 7759 2999
Fax: +44 20 7759 2901

Publisher: Andrew Ward
In-house editors: James Griffin and Catherine Harris
Design and artwork: AS&K Skylight Creative Services

ISBN-13: 978 1 901346 68 4
ISBN-10: 1 901346 68 4
British Library Cataloguing-in-Publication Data
A catalogue record for this book is available from the British Library.

Responsible Research

A GUIDE FOR COORDINATORS

Senior Editor

Carol A Fedor, ND, RN, CCRC
Clinical Research Manager
Center for Clinical Research
University Hospitals of Cleveland
Cleveland, Ohio, USA

Editors

Philip A Cola, MA
Director, Center for Clinical Research
University Hospitals of Cleveland
Cleveland, Ohio, USA

Christine Pierre, RN
President
Rx Trials, Inc.
Silver Spring, Maryland, USA

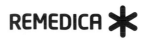

Contributors

Jean Booth, BSc, MSc, RGN
Senior Research Coordinator
Clinical Trials and Evaluation Unit
Royal Brompton and Harefield NHS Trust
Sydney Street
London SW3 6NP, UK

Philip A Cola, MA
Director, Center for Clinical Research
University Hospitals of Cleveland
11100 Euclid Avenue
Cleveland, OH 44106-7061, USA

Eric M Cottington, PhD
Associate Vice President for Research
Case Western Reserve University
Office of Sponsored Projects Administration
10900 Euclid Avenue
Cleveland, OH 44106-7015, USA

Barbara J Daly, PhD, RN, FAAN
Associate Professor
Case Western Reserve University
Director, Clinical Ethics
University Hospitals of Cleveland
11100 Euclid Avenue
Cleveland, OH 44106-7061, USA

Susan Davie
Unit Manager
Clinical Pharmacology
Australian Paediatric Pharmacology Research Unit
Royal Children's Hospital and Murdoch Children's Research Institute
Flemington Road
Parkville VIC 3052, Australia

Nicola Delahunty
Clinical Research Coordinator
Clinical Trials and Evaluation Unit
Royal Brompton and Harefield NHS Trust
Sydney Street
London SW3 6NP, UK

Carol A Fedor, ND, RN, CCRC
Clinical Research Manager
Center for Clinical Research
University Hospitals of Cleveland
11100 Euclid Avenue
Cleveland, OH 44106-7061, USA

Edward F Gabriele, DMin
Distinguished Faculty
Symposium Program Director
Society of Research Administrators International
1901 North Moore Street
Arlington, VA 22209, USA

Aviva Grosbard
Coordinator for Clinical Trials
Soroka University Medical Centre
Beer Sheva, Israel

Paula Jones-Wright, BScN, MEd, CCRC, CCRA
President
ClinCoach Inc.
12 Queen Street, Suite 204
Dartmouth, Nova Scotia
Canada B2Y 1E7

Felix A Khin-Maung-Gyi, PharmD, MBA, CIP
CEO, Co-founder
Chesapeake Research Review, Inc.
7063 Columbia Gateway Drive, Suite 110
Columbia, MD 21046-3403, USA

Belinda Lees, BSc, PhD
Senior Clinical Research Coordinator
Clinical Trials and Evaluation Unit
Royal Brompton and Harefield NHS Trust
Sydney Street
London SW3 6NP, UK

Rebecca Mister
Senior Clinical Research Coordinator
NHMRC Clinical Trials Centre
University of Sydney
88 Mallett Street
Camperdown, NSW 2050, Australia

Andrea G Procaccino, CCRT, CMT
Director, Technical Training
Master Certified Training Director
Johnson & Johnson Pharmaceutical Research & Development, LLC
1125 Trenton-Harbourton Road
Titusville, NJ 08560, USA

Matthew Whalen, PhD
President, Co-founder
Chesapeake Research Review, Inc.
7063 Columbia Gateway Drive, Suite 110
Columbia, MD 21046-3403, USA

Preface

"In general terms, responsible conduct in research is simply good citizenship applied to professional life."

An Introduction to the Responsible Conduct of Research

Office of Research Integrity

The concept for this book emerged from a feature series in the journal *Clinical Researcher* called 'The Coordinators' Forum'. I responded to an editorial in that journal, which commented on the immeasurable value of clinical research coordinators (CRCs). I approached the editor to suggest offering regular articles dedicated to CRCs. I eventually found myself overseeing that effort, which literally and figuratively opened up a whole new perspective on clinical research for me. After the first few articles were published, subsequent topics were obtained from CRCs around the world, providing an international perspective on clinical research and, later, the foundation for this book. I was intrigued to find that the role of the CRC is similar worldwide.

Responsible Research: A Guide for Coordinators has been developed for both novice and experienced CRCs. The chapters and content have been chosen to embrace not only the practical aspects of research conduct (eg, regulatory requirements, obtaining informed consent, communication), but also more detailed ethical issues (eg, responsible research conduct, assent with children, the professional role of CRCs). My co-editors and I decided that it was critical to discuss these concepts from a broad international perspective that included approaches from the European Union, Japan, and Canada, as well as the United States, which is reflected in our international authorship. In our surveys of CRCs, we have found that, irrespective of the particular research setting, the successful functioning of a clinical research team revolves around the CRC. Yet, there is remarkable inconsistency in CRCs' learning experiences, despite the availability of training and accreditation from professional organizations.

The editors and authors of this book were selected because of their hands-on experience with clinical research, as well as for their passion about the importance of personal contribution to the conduct of research. CRCs are said to be the "heart and soul" of clinical research. Hence, the quote at the beginning of this Preface reminds us that the quality of clinical research is only as good as the professionals who conduct it. The norms for responsible conduct vary from profession to profession, and thus we have developed this text, dedicated to CRCs, to offer a basis for understanding and conducting clinical research responsibly and with integrity.

Carol A Fedor
Senior Editor

Foreword

Clinical research, once considered primarily a scientific pursuit for academic medical centers, evolved over the past decade to what many saw as primarily a business activity. In contrast to the Fuller Albright model of investigational medicine, clinical trials were increasingly viewed as little more than the final common pathway for bringing a new drug, device, or biologic to market, and they frequently attracted more interest from investors than from scientists or physicians. Much of this evolution occurred rapidly during the early 90s during a period of rapid growth and intense competition among pharmaceutical and device companies. The desire, indeed, the competitive necessity, of being first-to-market with a new product placed a very real premium on speed at every stage of the clinical trials process, and many sponsors found that speed was not characteristic of traditional academic research sites.

I recall well attending a meeting about streamlining the clinical trials process while I was the Director of Clinical Research Support and Development at the Massachusetts General Hospital, listening to the CEO of a major contract research organization tell the audience that academic investigators were too arrogant and too slow, and that the performance of premier academic institutions in clinical research was inversely proportional to their reputations. At the same meeting, the word on the street was that the only good IRB was a fast IRB. Enrollment of subjects into trials emerged as the most valued feature of a research site, and those sites were rarely at a university medical center. They were physician offices and private research sites, and the 'investigators' were more often than not individuals with little or no experience or training in research, clinical or otherwise.

Looking back on the evolution of the clinical trials process from an academy-based scientific model to an industrial model, one can see the seeds for many of the challenges and opportunities, as well as problems facing clinical research today, and there are many. Financial incentives give rise to competing interests, and competitive performance pressures have led some to misconduct. Concerns about the safety and well being of research participants have taken center stage, with a caged "human guinea pig" prominently gracing the cover of *Time* magazine. Public trust in the process has eroded, we're told, and the Congress is considering sweeping legislation to fix the Food and Drug Administration. The sense of being in crisis is widespread, and calls for reform are loud and frequent.

And yet, against this backdrop of concern, one emergent group of clinical research professionals seems to have stayed above the fray, the clinical research coordinator, commonly referred to simply as research coordinators or CRCs.

Today, whether clinical research is done in an academic center, a physician's office, or a private site, the uniform key to quality work is a well-trained, committed professional research coordinator. Twenty years ago there was no such profession. Sure, there were secretaries and nurses working with physicians engaged in clinical trials, but there was no 'profession' as a research coordinator. Today there is, and its members are essential to responsible conduct of high-quality clinical research.

A profession, as characterized by Justice Louis Brandeis, is a group of individuals who have mastered a defined set of knowledge and possess specialized skills in an area of expertise for which it sets standards for practice and conduct. Professionals are generally focused on the services they provide and not primarily on the monetary aspects of their endeavors. Over the past 25 years, professionalization of the practice of research coordinators has been ongoing, including widespread certification by objective examination. This certification has become recognized by all who participate in clinical research, and is particularly valued by industrial sponsors of clinical research, where the rule of thumb is "no coordinator, no study!"

In this volume, Carol Fedor, Philip Cola, and Christine Pierre, three long-time leaders of the profession, have assembled an impressive collection of papers by knowledgeable experts encompassing the knowledge base that the professional coordinator is expected to master. Importantly, the approach taken is not focused on simple compliance with regulatory requirements, but instead focused on how a clinical research program should be managed by a responsible coordinator committed to the highest standards of performance, conduct, and protections for research participants. In taking this approach, the editors set a high standard for their colleagues already engaged in the profession, as well as for those newcomers just entering the field. In doing so, they serve their profession very well. Indeed, physician investigators would benefit from mastering the material covered herein, as the responsibility for professionalism in conducting clinical trials is shared.

At a time when the entire clinical trials process is facing challenges that have arisen both from its past and from our immense hope for a bright future, it is more important than ever that we all "do the right thing because it is the right thing to do." Continuing development of high-quality educational tools for a profession that continues to expand the scope and importance of its contributions to the successful clinical research endeavor is critical. The present effort is an exemplary step in the right direction.

Greg Koski, PhD, MD, CPI
Institute for Health Policy
Massachusetts General Hospital
Harvard Medical School

Former Director, Office for Human Research Protections
US Department of Health and Human Services

Contents

Chapter 1

The Evolving Role of the Clinical Research Coordinator

Carol A Fedor

Introduction

The development of new or improved treatments for debilitating conditions and diseases that affect people worldwide depends on the safe and competent conduct of clinical research. Clinical research promotes the understanding of these conditions and current methods of treatment, with the goal of more and better treatments for patients in the future.

Clinical research refers to the study of drugs, biologics, or devices in human subjects, with the intent of discovering beneficial effects and/or determining safety and efficacy [1]. Clinical research studies are designed to evaluate the safety and efficacy of investigational compounds, and they represent the fundamental process for bringing new therapies to market.

The recent growth in funding for biomedical research and consumer demand for access to new approved products has resulted in a substantial increase in the number of clinical trials initiated each year [2]. In the USA alone, increased investment in clinical research, by industry and/or federal funding, has resulted in an increase in the number of clinical trials: from 7,000 in 1990 to over 15,000 in 1997 [3]. These trends have resulted in the "emergence of an occupational group, research coordinators, devoted to overseeing the implementation of clinical trial protocols" [4].

There does not appear to be a distinct past event that marked the emergence of clinical trial coordination. However, the last 30 years have seen the realization of the clinical research profession, with the appearance of professional organizations for clinical researchers and publications describing the role of clinical research coordinators (CRCs). The profession of CRC evolved earlier in the USA than in the EU and Japan, but in these regions, and in Latin America, this recently established occupation is rapidly being formalized and advanced.

Clinical research studies are conducted by a qualified team of research staff, including CRCs, research/medical assistants, and data managers, and the research team is overseen by a principal investigator (PI), who is usually a physician. The PI serves as the team leader and is responsible for the professional conduct of the research, routinely assigning responsibilities to the study staff. The bulk of the clinical research study responsibilities are delegated to the CRC, who plays a multifaceted role in managing the study from start to finish.

The relationship between the PI, the CRC, and the entire research team is interdependent and is key to the success of a research study, so each team member must understand, respect, and support the others. The CRC "cannot successfully 'make the study happen' without the full support of the PI; likewise, the PI cannot maintain adequate control of the study without diligent attention from the CRC" [5].

Overview of the CRC's Responsibilities

Job Title
Depending on the type of research site where the study is being performed, there are diverse job titles that exist for the CRC role, including clinical research nurse, research coordinator, clinical trial coordinator, study coordinator, project manager, and data manager [4–8]. Regardless of the title, the CRC is under the immediate direction and supervision of the PI, and is compelled to ensure that research activities are conducted according to the regulatory guidelines. By far the most essential role fulfilled by the CRC is to protect the safety and well-being of the research participants.

Diverse Backgrounds

Based on the literature, a high percentage of CRCs have a nursing background [8–11], although other health occupations might be appropriate, depending on the therapeutic area of the clinical trial. The professional training and discipline of nurses are well-suited to the nature of the duties and responsibilities of the CRC, given nurses' understanding of medical interventions and procedures, patient-based assessments, informed consent, monitoring of adverse reactions, medical terminology and documentation, and the ethics of patient advocacy. Mueller and Mamo found that: "Nurses often sought out clinical research coordination in part because of the proximity of the career line to the work practices and skills in research" [2].

According to a *Clinical Researcher* survey, most often, "the CRC is a nurse who is experienced in a specific therapeutic disease area... who then gains knowledge about the responsible conduct of research from investigators and/or other qualified research professionals and administrators" [9]. In an editorial acknowledging CRCs as invaluable members of the research team, Dr Joseph Pergolizzi, Jr, reflected that "Today, things have changed, with the modern coordinator's role expanding beyond the realm of nursing. It could now be described as something of an eclectic position, involving individuals from diverse backgrounds, such as nutritionists and therapists. But while this transformation has brought many advantages, it has also contributed to the dilemma of properly defining the role and responsibilities of a coordinator" [12].

The Evolving Role of the CRC

To best interpret the evolving role of the CRC, it is essential to examine the scope of the responsibilities that CRCs perform. Initially, the role of the CRC related to the clinical management of the patient, or to aspects of nursing care under the auspices of an assistant to the physician. Over time, the role of the CRC has advanced to include more diverse and specialized functions, such as responsibility for recruitment, data, regulatory documentation, tracking of the financial status of the study, staff supervision, training and mentoring, evaluating the feasibility of new studies, and communicating with the institutional review board (IRB)/independent ethics commitee (IEC) and sponsor, as well as monitoring (see Table 1).

The Association of Clinical Research Professionals (ACRP) (see Table 2) provides the following definition of the CRC role: "A clinical research coordinator, study site

• Serving as the primary advocate for the research participant	• Overseeing investigational product accountability by liaising with the pharmacy, and monitoring research participants' compliance
• Initiating the informed consent process and ensuring that consent procedures are compliant with Good Clinical Practice	• Preparing the site for monitoring visits or other mandated audits
• Completing regulatory documents	• Completing study documentation (eg, case report forms, continuing ethics board reviews) in a timely manner in compliance with the regulations
• Creating and negotiating the study budget and assessing site costs	
• Preparing ethics committee submissions	
• Liaising with the study sponsor's representatives	• Maintaining a research record for each screened and enrolled research participant
• Facilitating communication and decision-making within the research team	• Maintaining the regulatory binder
• Networking and building referral mechanisms for subject recruitment	• Organizing storage and space requirements (eg, for records, the investigational product, specimen containers)
• Developing a strategic recruitment and retention plan	
• Coordinating and scheduling visit appointments and research team meetings	• Monitoring and reporting adverse events
	• Educating research participants and research team members
• Performing research assessments, collecting data, and confirming source documentation	• Keeping the research team motivated throughout the study
• Obtaining required specimens and vital signs according to the protocol	

Table 1. A summary of the main activities and responsibilities carried out by the clinical research coordinator. (Note: Sometimes these activities may be delegated to other members of the research team.)

research nurse or study site coordinator, [who] works at a clinical research site under the immediate direction of a principal investigator, whose research activities are conducted under Good Clinical Practice regulations. Among other tasks, CRCs perform site preparation, patient screening and recruitment, patient enrollment, conduct and ensure the quality of case report forms, maintain source documents, and ensure site quality" [13].

It has been said that the CRC is the heart and soul of the research study and that, ultimately, it is the CRC who carries forward the research goals, thereby playing a significant role in the success of the research study. Most importantly, CRCs are often involved in essential duties that have been traditionally performed by the PI, such as conducting the informed consent process and ensuring compliance with the protocol.

The ACRP, founded in 1976, is comprised of a diverse network of clinical research professionals including clinical research coordinators, investigators and associates, research and development project managers, regulatory affairs and compliance professionals, and quality control and assurance auditors. ACRP's membership spans 52 countries and includes more than 19,000 members. ACRP offers training classes and certification in both US Food and Drug Administration and International Conference on Harmonisation processes.

Table 2. The Association of Clinical Research Professionals (ACRP).

A significant percentage of the publications that describe the role of CRCs and research nurses are to be found in the oncology and nursing literature. The role of the CRC can be compared internationally through a survey that was distributed to 41 CRCs involved in oncology clinical trials in Spain. It was concluded that "CRCs are mainly devoted to monitoring activities including patient registration/ randomization, recruitment follow-up, case report form completion, collaboration with the CRA [clinical research associate], serious adverse event reporting, investigator file handling, and preparing the site for and/or attending audits" [6].

The survey results further delineated that "Nurses and physicians had greater involvement in clinical activities, such as completion of scales/questionnaires... response to therapy assessment... and toxicity assessment"[6]. In addition, query resolution was performed by 100% of CRCs with a nurse/physician background compared with 60.9% of CRCs with a different background. Of note, 74.3% of the respondents to the survey held the title 'data managers' while only 8.6% held the title 'clinical research coordinator'.

Variations in Responsibilities

The multifaceted responsibilities of the CRC described in the literature are similar regardless of the therapeutic area or geographic region [5,6,9,14,15]. For example, in The Netherlands, "Research nurses [ie, CRCs] can fill many roles in clinical research: direct care provider, educator, coordinator, data collector, researcher, [and] team member. Regardless of the role, research nurses hold key positions with regards to supporting, guiding and motivating trial subjects and ensuring that trials are carried out with scientific and ethical integrity. In this, they are confronted with problems that can be divided into three main categories: decision-making, conflict between different responsibilities, and ethical and moral problems" [15].

The complex duties that CRCs must carry out might vary to some extent, depending on the type of research being conducted, the environment in which the research is conducted, and the cultural influences driving the regulations governing clinical research. Nevertheless, it is unequivocal that the foremost responsibilities of the CRC are:

- advocacy for research participants
- ensuring the responsible conduct of the study

It is necessary to balance these roles throughout the study, beginning with protocol development, recruitment, screening, and enrollment.

The *caring* provided by the CRC must integrate the *realism* of research – or, as summarized by Davis et al., "Responding to the hopeful subject, as patient advocates [CRCs] want to encourage patients' hope but not take advantage of it. As study advocates, [CRCs] recognize the value of hope in encouraging subject participation; and as subject advocates, they move away from both of those positions to one of neutrality, providing information but without unduly influencing decision-making" [8]. Indeed, it is the CRC who is particularly involved with protection of the research participant and who routinely faces challenging ethical issues, a fact that points to the need for recognition by professional organizations and regulatory agencies that a core educational requirement for CRCs should be training in research ethics and the responsible conduct of research.

Training and Certification

While the role of care provider is one of the foremost activities involved in clinical trials, to manage the full spectrum of research activities CRCs require a wide range of technical, managerial, ethical, and regulatory expertise. According to an interview-based study of 32 nurses and clinical trial coordinators [11], none had received formal course instruction on clinical trials as part of their basic nursing training and the nurses "learned about clinical research 'on the job', initially through an orientation provided by the investigator or by another coordinator".

The value of adequate training in clinical research and principles of Good Clinical Practice is consistently reported by authors [6,9,14], as well-trained and experienced CRCs contribute significantly to the quality of data collected and promote the responsible conduct of research. ACRP offers a CRC certification (CCRC) in recognition of:

- documented and verified work experience; and
- successful performance in a multiple-choice exam

The credential of CCRC identifies the standard of practice for clinical research coordinators. The 2003 ACRP member survey discovered that certification is encouraged by 50% of employers and that it has a positive impact on salary [16]. Since 1992, ACRP has certified over 9,500 clinical research coordinators.

CRC Workload and Turnover

Over the past three years, several surveys have revealed the following insights into CRC workload:

- In 2002, a CenterWatch survey indicated that CRC workload (measured by the number of clinical trials actively managed by each CRC) was rising by 6% per year, with an average of 4.3 trials per CRC [17].
- Another survey conducted in 2003 found that CRCs manage about five studies each, and thus do a lot of multitasking.
- In 2004, CenterWatch reported that CRC workload had intensified further due to the implementation of electronic data capture, and increased adverse event and regulatory reporting [18].

Based on these trends, it is no surprise that the rate of staff turnover is increasing.

It is unfortunate that, according to anecdotal evidence, CRCs often leave their position for a higher paying position of monitor (the role of the monitor is discussed in **Chapter 10**). However, many CRCs remain in their position due to personal and professional satisfaction. To retain CRCs, research sites are incorporating incentives such as increased salary levels, improved benefits packages, flexible hours, hiring of additional staff to assist with regulatory and recruitment requirements, and opportunities for promotions and career advancement. In order to influence the CRC turnover rate, job satisfaction must be nurtured at the research site, by providing opportunities for growth and professional development, as well as continuous recognition of CRCs' accomplishments.

Compensation

According to the 2003 ACRP survey [16], the following salary trends were identified for CRCs:

- Most CRC positions (68%) are salaried, while others (30%) are paid hourly. The salaried positions are predominantly full-time.
- A typical full-time CRC will earn US$50,000 in basic salary. Variations in salary tend to be based on factors such as number of staff, years of experience, education, and type of site.
- Certification credentials have a definite impact on salary, although not all certifications are recognized by an increased salary. CRCs holding a CCRC report a median salary of US$50,000, whereas those not holding certification report a median salary of US$45,000.
- One-third of the full-time, salaried CRCs reported receiving a cash bonus in 2002.

Skills and Characteristics Required by CRCs

The CRC role varies depending on the type of research being conducted and the site profile. However, standardization of the job description will result in a more realistic determination of CRC workload. Certain responsibilities that are time intensive or require expertise, such as recruitment and completing regulatory or IRB/IEC documentation, might be delegated to a designated team member to maximize the efficiency of the team. The essential characteristics of the CRC are listed in **Table 3**.

Conclusion

The role of the CRC has grown in its sophistication over the past 30 years and currently involves a more in-depth and specialized knowledge base than ever before. CRCs not only perform the everyday tasks essential to the conduct of the study, but are also involved in compliance, research administration, marketing, and fiscal and legal activities. The role of the CRC may vary depending on the type of research being conducted and the site profile, but a realistic determination of the CRC's

• Attention to detail when documenting data in research records	• Adherence to standards, regulations, and instructions
• Ability to deal professionally with research participants and act as their advocate	• An understanding of ethical issues and issues of potential conflict of interest
• Ability to work independently and as a team with the principal investigator and other research staff	• An understanding of the drug development process
• Knowledge of Good Clinical Practice and country-specific regulations	• An understanding of the legal and fiscal requirements of the study
• Good project management skills	• The ability to lead a team and be a mentor
• Deadline oriented	• Strong interpersonal skills
• Initiative and self-motivational ability	• Responsible

Table 3. Essential characteristics of a clinical research coordinator.

workload is essential in order to preserve the integrity of the research. Certain responsibilities that are time intensive or require specific expertise, such as recruitment and completing regulatory or ethics committee documentation, should be assigned to a suitable team member to take advantage of the variety of skills of the research team.

It is widely accepted that CRCs are of vital importance in clinical research studies, and sponsors and contract research organizations increasingly acknowledge that a strong CRC is essential to ensuring the success of a study. The success of the research study depends on diligence, creative problem-solving, and hard work. At long last, CRCs are receiving the respect and recognition they deserve for their historic contribution to the responsible conduct of clinical research.

References

1. Dunn C, Chadwick G. Protecting Study Volunteers in Research. A Manual for Investigative Sites. Boston, MA: CenterWatch, Inc., 1999:219.

2. Mueller MR, Mamo L. Changes in medicine, changes in nursing: career contingencies of nurses into clinical trial coordination. Sociol Perspect 2000;43(4):S43-57.

3. Flaherty M. Search for answers: drug trials create ethical balancing act. Nurse Week 1999;12(1):14.

4. Mueller MR, Mamo L. The nurse clinical trial coordinator: benefits and drawbacks of the role. Res Theory Nurs Pract 2002;16(1):33-42.

5. Pelke S, Easa D. The role of the clinical research coordinator in multicenter clinical trials. J Obstet Gynecol Neonatal Nurs 1997;26(3):279-85.

6. Rico-Villademoros F, Hernando T, Sanz J-L, et al. The role of the clinical research coordinator – data manager – in oncology clinical trials. BMC Med Res Methodol 2004;4:6.

7. Kellen JC, Schron EB, McBride R, et al. A survey of clinical trial coordinators: factors influencing job satisfaction and turnover. Cardiovasc Nurs 1994;30(4):25-31.

8. Davis AM, Hull SC, Grady C, et al. The invisible hand in clinical research: the study coordinator's critical role in human subjects protection. J Law Med Ethics 2002;30(3):411-9.

9. Fedor C, Cola P. Preliminary results of the Clinical Researcher coordinators' survey. Clinical Researcher 2003;3(4):18-22.

10. Halloran L. ACRP's North American salary analysis. The Monitor 1998;Winter.

11. Mueller MR. From delegation to specialization: nurses and clinical trial coordination. Nurs Inq 2001;8(3):182-90.

12. Pergolizzi J. The changing role of the modern coordinator. Clinical Researcher 2001;1(2):4-5.

13. Certification Exam Review Courses for CRAs and CRCs [web page]. Available from: www.acrpnet.org/ education/examrev/index.html. Accessed November 15, 2004.

14. Arrigo C, Gall H, Delogne A, et al. The involvement of nurses in clinical trials: results of the EORTC Oncology Nurses Study Group survey. Cancer Nurs 1994;17(5):429-33.

15. Kragt K, Bruggeling MM, Huisman AJ, et al. Research nurses in The Netherlands are profiled based on responses to two surveys. Applied Clinical Trials 2001;10(6):100.

16. ACRP. 2003 Compensation and Benefits Survey. Final Report. Alexandra, VA: ACRP, 2003.

17. Neuer A. The rising tide of CRC workload and turnover. CenterWatch 2002;9(8);1-7.

18. Borfitz D. CRC loss tied to heavy workload. CenterWatch 2004;11(8):1-6.

Chapter 2

Guiding Principles and Regulations

Paula Jones-Wright

Introduction

There are many sets of guidelines and regulations in place around the world to govern clinical research. These rules and guidances take many forms, such as specifying steps to ensure the accurate collection and presentation of data, but all are based around ethical principles that state that research participants must not be subjected to any unnecessary risk during a study.

As a clinical research coordinator (CRC), it is essential for you to be aware of, and understand, all of the rules and regulations that apply in your region – and, in the case of multicenter trials, those that apply in other countries as well. It is also now important for you to know the rules that are in place for tackling the relatively new concept of protecting personal health information.

Of course, it is one thing to know and understand the guidelines and regulations, but it is another challenge to ensure that they are followed. The best way to make certain that clinical research is performed correctly is to create standard operating procedures (SOPs) for all site staff to follow, and to ensure that everyone is properly trained. This chapter outlines the major guidelines and regulations that you need to know, and explains how they should be implemented to help to ensure that your clinical research is safe and efficient.

Country	Regulation
USA	Food and Drug Administration Code of Federal Regulations
EU	Clinical Trials Directive
Canada	Health Canada Therapeutic Products Directorate's Food and Drug Regulations for Clinical Trials

Table 1. Examples of clinical research regulations.

Guidelines versus Regulations

Before going into the specifics of any of the main clinical research guidelines and regulations, it is worth pointing out the conceptual difference between guidelines and regulations. Simply speaking, every standard in professional practice generally begins as a guideline. As standards become adopted internationally by individual countries they become national regulations – legal standards – that must be followed (see **Table 1**).

Guidelines only give guidance to researchers, but must be followed as strictly as regulations because they represent standards in practice that should be maintained. While breaching them is not in itself punishable by law, failure to comply can have disciplinary consequences or can lead to legal liability through, for example, breach of study protocol, breach of SOPs, or negligence to participants.

Ultimately, the failure to comply with guidelines could invalidate a study, meaning that participants would have been exposed to needless risks (because the data obtained from such as study would be invalid, making all study procedures unnecessary), and resulting in the failure of the site in the eyes of the sponsor, with all of the associated repercussions.

Therefore, as a CRC it is essential that you follow all of the applicable guidelines and regulations, at all times. Because the consequences of failing to do so are so serious, you must ensure that you are well informed of your legal liabilities in clinical research practice – this involves a detailed assessment of whether your qualifications and skills meet the required standards for the clinical research you are involved in. Be warned: CRCs can be liable for human subject noncompliance and/or scientific misconduct if the guidelines and regulations are not strictly respected.

In Canada, the document that describes the ethical standards and procedures for research involving human subjects is a guideline called the "Tricouncil Policy Statement: Ethical Conduct for Research Involving Humans", which has been in use since 1998 [1]. This document promotes the ethical conduct of research involving human subjects, and is implemented by the research ethics boards in Canada. Of particular interest for clinical research coordinators are Section 2, which relates to informed consent, and Section 7, which relates to clinical trials.

Table 2. The implementation of guidelines: Canada.

Ethical Foundations

Ethical principles provide clear moral foundations for guidelines and regulations. In **Chapter 3**, ethics and human subjects protection are discussed in more detail, and a concise summary is provided of the key ethical documents that have contributed to modern clinical research guidelines and regulations.

Essentially, the crux of these principles is that the health and welfare of research participants should not be compromised by involvement in research. Guidelines have been created that suggest ways of working that are compatible with these principles. National regulations have then been drawn up by adapting the most important parts of these guidelines and adding supplementary information to fit in with the customs and cultures of the country. This means that a guideline will be implemented in different ways in different countries (see **Table 2**).

International Guidelines

The central international guidelines for clinical research conduct are the International Conference on Harmonisation guidelines for Good Clinical Practice (ICH–GCP). It is vital for all CRCs to understand these guidelines as ICH–GCP is a template for Good Clinical Practice (GCP) worldwide, and most major clinical research regions have used it as the basis for their national regulations. Before looking at the specifics of ICH–GCP, it is useful to look at how and why it was produced, and its scope.

The International Conference on Harmonisation

In April 1990, the ICH, or, to give it its full title, the "International Conference on Harmonisation of the Technical Requirements for the Registration of

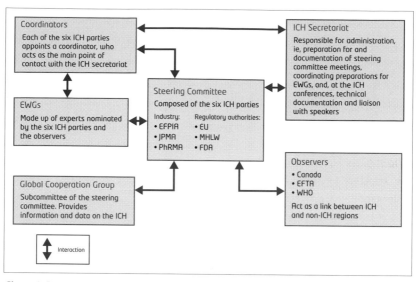

Figure 1. Structure of the International Conference on Harmonisation (ICH) [9]. EFPIA: European Federation of Pharmaceutical Industries and Associations; EFTA: European Free Trade Association; EWG: expert working group; FDA: US Food and Drug Administration; JPMA: Japan Pharmaceutical Manufacturers Association; MHLW: Japanese Ministry of Health, Labor, and Welfare; PhRMA: Pharmaceutical Research and Manufacturers of America; WHO: World Health Organization.

Pharmaceuticals for Human Use," was established with the aim of globally harmonizing every step in pharmaceutical research and development. The ICH's stated terms of reference are [2]:

- to maintain a forum for constructive dialogue between regulatory authorities and the pharmaceutical industry on the real and perceived differences in the technical requirements for product registration in the EU, USA, and Japan in order to ensure a more timely introduction of new medicinal products, and their availability to patients
- to contribute to the protection of public health from an international perspective
- to monitor and update harmonized technical requirements, leading to a greater mutual acceptance of research and development data
- to avoid divergent future requirements through harmonization of selected topics needed as a result of therapeutic advances and the development of new technologies for the production of medicinal products

- to facilitate the adoption of new or improved technical research and development approaches that update or replace current practices, where these permit a more economical use of human, animal, and material resources, without compromising safety
- to facilitate the dissemination and communication of information on harmonized guidelines and their use such as to encourage the implementation and integration of common standards

Who makes the decisions?

The structure of the ICH is fairly complex (see **Figure 1**), but it is worth understanding (see Reference 9 for an overview).

The steering committee of the ICH is the decision-making heart of the organization. It exists to determine the policies and procedures of the ICH, select topics for harmonization, and monitor the progress of harmonization initiatives. It meets at least twice a year. It is made up of six directly involved parties:

- EU
- European Federation of Pharmaceutical Industries and Associations
- Japanese Ministry of Health, Labor, and Welfare
- Japan Pharmaceutical Manufacturers Association
- US Food and Drug Administration (FDA)
- Pharmaceutical Research and Manufacturers of America

All six parties come from three regions – Europe, USA, and Japan – reflecting the areas in which the harmonization process was started. Other countries are also involved, albeit at a different level for now. There are three ICH observers, which are bodies acting as a link between the ICH and non-ICH regions. They are:

- Health Canada
- World Health Organization
- European Free Trade Association

In addition, the International Federation of Pharmaceutical Manufacturers Associations is designated as the ICH secretariat. It is responsible for the administration of everything the ICH does, such as preparing and documenting meetings.

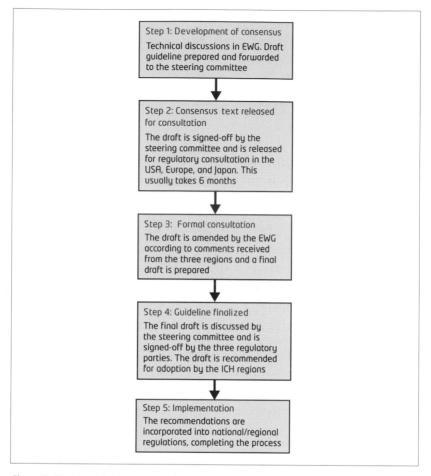

Figure 2. The harmonization process of the International Conference on Harmonisation [9]. EWG: expert working group.

The last major component of the ICH involves expert working groups (EWGs), which are formed for each technical topic selected for harmonization. Each EWG reviews the differences between the three regions and develops a scientific consensus regarding the harmonization of its topic. EWGs comprise scientific and regulatory experts from ICH steering committee and observer countries: the experts can be representatives from the pharmaceutical industry, the self-medication industry, or the generic industry.

How are guidelines made?

The ICH has four main categories of guidelines:

- quality (Q)
- safety (S)
- efficacy (E)
- multidisciplinary (M)

In total, more than 60 guidelines have been produced. The process of harmonizing a particular aspect of the registration of pharmaceuticals is a multistep process (see **Figure 2**).

First, the need for harmonization of a specific aspect is identified by one or more of the ICH parties, who then become the 'sponsors' for the topic. The sponsors submit a proposal to the steering committee, which then decides, over the course of several meetings, whether to include the topic in the ICH process. If the steering committee decides to proceed with the proposal, it forms an EWG, which then meets and gathers ideas (*step 1*).

A set of draft guidelines is then written (a *step 2* document) and is submitted to the steering committee for sign-off by the six ICH parties. This document is then released to the three ICH regions for a consultation period of about 6 months.

All comments are then considered by the EWG, which then draws up a final draft of the guidelines (*step 3*). This final draft is then endorsed by the steering committee and signed-off by the three regulatory parties, and is recommended for adoption in the ICH regions (*step 4*).

The final step – *step 5* – occurs when the ICH regions incorporate the guidelines into national regulations.

The Good Clinical Practice Guideline

ICH–GCP, classified as efficacy guideline E6, was officially adopted by the EU in 1996, and by Japan and the USA in 1997, although this does not, as described earlier, mean that it has become legally enforceable in these territories. The guideline outlines requirements for designing, conducting, recording, and reporting trials that involve the participation of human subjects. Compliance with this standard achieves two goals:

- It provides public assurance that the rights, safety, and wellbeing of trial subjects are protected, consistent with the ethical principles that have their origin in the "Declaration of Helsinki".
- It ensures that the clinical trial data obtained from a study will meet the requirements of the regulatory authorities in the EU, Japan, and the USA.

It is encouraging to know that ICH–GCP is also being used by trial sponsors and research staff in many non-ICH countries, eg, in developing countries such as those in Africa.

The principles established in this guideline can also be applied to other clinical investigations that may have an impact on the safety and wellbeing of human subjects, eg, natural products research and general academic research that would not traditionally be considered a clinical trial. In fact, from my own experience as a clinical research trainer, I have found that many of the researchers conducting clinical research that is not sponsored by drug companies (eg, nutraceutical research) are now seeing the benefits of complying with ICH–GCP and are implementing it in their clinical practice.

The CRC's Responsibilities

Although the role and responsibilities of the CRC are not mentioned by name in ICH–GCP, the fact that many principal investigators (PIs) delegate tasks to CRCs means that you must be familiar with section 4 of ICH–GCP, entitled "Investigator" [2]. The responsibilities of the PI, and guidelines regarding audits and monitoring visits, are all listed in ICH–GCP; these can be a good source of information about monitoring visits.

While it is the PI who is specified as the responsible party, the CRC should understand the principles of ICH–GCP. This allows the PI to be confident that all delegates are capable of conducting the necessary tasks, and helps you to help the PI to achieve the goals that he/she is responsible for. It is particularly important for the CRC to know and understand the following ICH–GCP principles that sites must comply with.

Rights and Safety of Human Subjects

"The rights, safety, and wellbeing of trial subjects are the most important considerations and should prevail over interests of science and society" [2].

Risk to Benefit Ratio
"Before a trial is initiated, the foreseeable risks and inconveniences should be weighed against the anticipated benefit for the individual trial subject and society" [2].

This evaluation should be done before a clinical trial is initiated by the sponsor and the institutional review board (IRB)/independent ethics committee (IEC) reviews the research. A clinical trial should be initiated and continued only if the anticipated benefits justify the risks: understanding this concept will help you when preparing IRB/IEC submissions.

Investigator's Brochure
The investigator's brochure must contain adequate clinical and nonclinical information on the investigational product to support the proposed clinical trial. The purpose of the investigator's brochure is to allow members of the research team to understand the rationale for the study and how to comply with the protocol.

The adequacy of the information in the investigator's brochure is determined by the regulatory body (eg, FDA) when the sponsor seeks approval for the clinical trial. For example, if permission is sought for a Phase I study, all data from preclinical research must be submitted; the adequacy of this information is then determined by experts who decide whether to allow the trial to go ahead. Such data is sent to the site for review by the PI and the CRC, and will form the basis of the product monograph should the drug be approved.

Protocol
"Clinical trials should be scientifically sound and described in a clear, detailed protocol" [2].

A trial should be conducted in compliance with a protocol that has received prior IRB/IEC approval/favorable opinion. A protocol allows the study team less personal judgment than medical practice – it must be followed to the letter or, if amendments are made, they must be approved by the IRB/IEC.

Qualifications and Training
"Each individual involved in conducting a trial should be qualified by education, training, and experience to perform his or her respective task(s)" [2].

Sponsors and university research sites should recognize both the need for training clinical research team members and the documentation of this training.

> In the USA, clinical nurse practitioners can become investigators, although this is usually with the involvement of a physician or dentist as coinvestigator. In Canada, the regulations state that only a licensed physician or dentist can be an investigator, and that nurses and nonmedical doctors (ie, those with a PhD) cannot.

Table 3. Who can be considered as an investigator?

Subjects' Medical Care

"The medical care given to, and medical decisions made on behalf of, subjects should always be the responsibility of a qualified physician or, when appropriate, a qualified dentist" [2].

The interpretation of this principle varies slightly depending on the country (see **Table 3**).

Informed Consent

"Freely given informed consent should be obtained from every subject prior to clinical trial participation" [2].

Informed consent is an ongoing process throughout the trial and the participant is free to withdraw from research at any time, for whatever reason. The informed consent process is examined in more detail in **Chapter 5**.

Good Manufacturing Practice

"Investigational products should be manufactured, handled, and stored in accordance with applicable Good Manufacturing Practice. They should be used in accordance with the approved protocol" [2].

Shipping of the investigational product must be done in accordance with the protocol and other rules, such as those of the International Air Transport Association. The clinical trial pharmacist (if used by the site) plays a vital role in assuring investigational product compliance. For smaller sites, the CRC might be expected to take on the role of pharmacist for the study.

Documentation

"All clinical trial information should be recorded, handled, and stored in a way that allows its accurate reporting, interpretation, and verification" [2].

Documentation is discussed in detail in **Chapter 9**.

Confidentiality

"The confidentiality of records that could identify subjects should be protected, respecting the privacy and confidentiality rules in accordance with the applicable regulatory requirement(s)" [2].

This is examined in more detail later in this chapter.

Quality Procedures

Systems of procedures should be implemented to assure the quality of every aspect of the trial. SOPs can be used to ensure that this general GCP responsibility is met. The role of the clinical research associate (monitor) also ensures that the aspects of quality assurance and quality control are implemented sufficiently. This is discussed further in **Chapter 10**.

Country-specific Regulations

As well as following ICH–GCP, it is vitally important for you to understand and comply with the guidelines and regulations that apply in the region in which you are working. While ICH–GCP is valid globally and has been adopted by many countries as the basis for their national clinical research standards, the key territories of the EU and the USA have enacted legislation to make the main aspects of ICH–GCP legally enforceable. **Table 4** outlines the bodies that enforce clinical research regulations and compile guidance within these regions.

The USA
The Department of Health and Human Services (HHS)

In the USA, HHS is the government's principle agency for protecting the health of all Americans. It is the grant-making agency, providing 60,000 grants per year. It comprises several public health service agencies, including the FDA and the National Institutes of Health (NIH) (see below).

The Food and Drug Administration

The FDA is the main legislative body in the USA in terms of clinical research regulations. It maintains the Code of Federal Regulations (CFR), which is the overall regulatory document regarding all aspects of FDA policy. Title 21 CFR contains the rules applicable to CRCs (see **Table 5** for a summary) [4]. CFR is generally consistent with ICH–GCP, but contains additional details on such issues

Region	Body	Description	Regulations/guidelines	Further information
USA	HHS	Made up of FDA and NIH	As detailed for FDA and NIH	www.os.dhhs.gov
	FDA	Protects the public health by assuring the safety, and efficacy and security of human and veterinary drugs, biological products, medical devices, the USA's food supply, cosmetics, and products that emit radiation	Maintains the CFR, which are legally enforceable rules regarding, among other issues, the conduct of clinical research	www.fda.gov
		Is the body that pharmaceutical marketing/ registration studies must be submitted to		
	NIH	Aims to achieve better health for everyone	OHRP - oversight function Common rule (45 CFR 46)	www.nih.gov
		Conducts research in its own laboratories		
		Supports the research of non-federal scientists in universities, medical schools, hospitals, and research institutions throughout the country and abroad		
		Helps train research investigators		
		Fosters communication of medical information		
EU	EC	Operates at the very heart of the EU	Responsible for the European Directives and Regulations on clinical research	europa.eu.int/ comm/index_ en.htm
		Proposes legislation to the Council of the EU and European Parliament		
		Manages the implementation of EU legislation by working with Member States and other European institutions		

Table 4. Regulatory bodies in the USA and EU. CFR: Code of Federal Regulations; EC: European Commission; EMEA: European Medicines Evaluation Agency; FDA: Food and Drug Administration; HHS: Department of Health and Human Services; ICH-GCP: International Conference on Harmonisation guidelines for Good Clinical Practice; NIH: National Institutes of Health; OHRP: Office of Human Research Protections.

Region	Body	Description	Regulations/guidelines	Further information
EU	EMEA	Protection and promotion of public and animal health	Oversight of ICH–GCP in EU countries	www.emea.eu.int
		Evaluation of medicinal products	Body to which registration studies are submitted for centralized EU approval	
		Provides information on medicines to users and health professionals		
		Single, centralized route for European marketing authorizations		
		Controls the safety of medicines for humans and animals, through a pharmacovigilance network		
		Establishes safe limits for residues in food-producing animals		

Table 4. Continued.

as electronic records (21 CFR 11) and human subjects protection (21 CFR 50), and also has requirements for financial disclosure (21 CFR 54), which is not covered in ICH–GCP.

The National Institutes of Health

The NIH is one of the world's leading medical research centers and acts as the country's federal focal point for medical research. The NIH is made up of 27 separate institutes and centers, which are part of the HHS. The goal of NIH research is "To acquire new knowledge to help prevent, detect, diagnose, and treat disease and disability, from the rarest genetic disorder to the common cold" [5]. The aim of the NIH is better health for everyone. The NIH recognizes and advocates implementation of ICH–GCP into clinical research practice.

The European Union

The EU currently includes the following 25 countries: Austria, Belgium, Denmark, Finland, France, Germany, Greece, Ireland, Italy, Luxembourg, The Netherlands, Portugal, Spain, Sweden, the UK, the Czech Republic, Estonia, Cyprus, Latvia, Lithuania, Hungary, Malta, Poland, Slovenia, and Slovakia. It is important for you to know which European countries are affected by EU guidelines and regulations.

Regulation	Topic	Notable subparts	Year implemented
21 CFR 11	Electronic records and signatures	–	1997
21 CFR 50	Protection of human subjects	B: informed consent D: additional safeguards for children	1980
21 CFR 54	Financial disclosure by investigators	–	1998
21 CFR 56	Institutional review boards	B: membership C: functions and operations	1981
21 CFR 312	Investigational new drug applications	D: responsibilities of sponsors and investigators F: foreign clinical studies not conducted under an investigational new drug application (312.120)	1987
21 CFR 314	Applications for FDA approval to market a new drug	D: acceptability of foreign data (314.106)	1985
21 CFR 601	Licensing biological products	–	1973
21 CFR 812	Investigational device exemptions	D: IRB review and approval E: responsibilities of investigators G: records and reports	1980
21 CFR 814	Premarket approval of medical devices	–	1986

Table 5. Sections of the Code of Federal Regulations (CFR) applicable to clinical research coordinators. (See Reference 3 for online versions of the various parts of CFR Title 21.) FDA: US Food and Drug Administration; IRB: institutional review board.

The EU consists of five institutions:

1. European Parliament
2. Council of the European Union
3. European Commission (EC)
4. Court of Justice
5. Court of Auditors

Of these, the EC is the most important for you to understand.

The European Commission

The EC is a politically independent institution that represents and upholds the interests of the EU as a whole. Two of its main functions are to propose legislation to the Council of the EU and the European Parliament, and to manage the implementation of EU legislation. The main EU directive of interest to CRCs is directive 2001/20/EC, the EU Clinical Trials Directive.

The Clinical Trials Directive came into force in May 2004. Following ICH–GCP, it is a further attempt to harmonize clinical research studies across the EU member states – it aims to provide a legal framework for the application of GCP to all trials conducted in the EU. All clinical research studies that involve medicinal products are covered by the Clinical Trials Directive, with the exception of noninterventional trials (eg, epidemiology studies). Member states are legally bound to use the harmonized principles of GCP covering the design, conduct, recording, and reporting of clinical research studies.

The European Medicines Evaluation Agency

The European Medicines Evaluation Agency (EMEA) is responsible for the protection and promotion of public and animal health throughout the EU. To achieve this, it mobilizes scientific resources from throughout the EU. The EMEA evaluates medicinal products, advises on research and development programs, controls the safety of medicines for humans and animals through a pharmacovigilance network, establishes safe limits for residues in food-producing animals, and provides information to the users of medicinal products and health professionals.

The EMEA is responsible for the oversight of ICH–GCP in EU countries, as well as being the body to which registration studies are submitted for central approval within the EU.

Privacy Legislation

Public privacy issues are becoming increasingly important in many areas of life, mainly due to the greater use of technology such as computer database systems. Healthcare information is one area in which many governments have decided to introduce legislation to protect the rights of patients and to limit the collection, use, and disclosure of patients' personal data. In the USA, such personal data are known as protected health information (PHI), while in Canada they are known as personal health information.

When taking part in clinical research, you should be accountable for the implementation of human subject data privacy and aware of local requirements regarding the protection of PHI. The health information you deal with is deemed to be highly sensitive, so confidentiality (as required by GCP) is crucial, along with respect for the participant's privacy in general.

General Principles

When conducting clinical research, you should consider the following questions regarding PHI [6–8]:

- What is the purpose of the research and what data are required to fulfill this objective(s)?
- What is the nature of the data that will be collected and analyzed, used, or disclosed?
- Are there any commercial aspects of the research activity?
- Does the research have any connection with the operation of a federal business?
- What is the geographic scope of the research?
- What is the general requirement for informed consent (ie, ICH–GCP)?
- What is the general requirement for privacy consent (ie, privacy rules)?
- What data-management practices are in place at the site?
- What is the potential long-term impact of these data-management practices on subjects' data?

US Regulations
Protected health information

In the USA, PHI is a subset of what is termed *individually identifiable health information* [8]. This is defined as information:

- concerning the physical or mental health of an individual
- concerning any health service provided to an individual
- concerning the donation by the individual of any body part or any bodily substance, or derived from the testing or examination of a body part or bodily substance of the individual

- that is collected in the course of providing health services to an individual
- that is collected incidentally to the provision of health services to an individual

The Health Insurance Portability and Accountability Act (HIPAA) – referred to as the Privacy Rule – was developed in 1996 by the HHS Office for Civil Rights, and came into force on April 14, 2003 [8]. The Privacy Rule places new conditions on the use and disclosure of PHI by covered entities for research.

A covered entity is defined as: "A health plan, a health care clearinghouse, or a health care provider who transmits any health information in electronic form in connection with a HIPAA transaction."

Authorization forms

In the USA, CRCs are responsible for ensuring compliance with HIPAA through the presentation of authorization forms to patients participating in clinical trials. Authorization is usually incorporated into the informed consent process, although in some studies a separate form will be required. You should inform the participant about who will have access to their PHI and why, and that the FDA might inspect their records. Authorizations should also include a time limit – either indefinite, or stating an appropriate end date (eg, database closure at the end of the study).

The authorization form gives the participant's signed permission for their PHI, as described in the authorization, to be used or disclosed for the purpose(s) and to the recipient(s) stated in the authorization. An exception to this is adverse event reporting. Even if a participant withdraws their authorization then you should continue to report adverse events to the sponsor. This helps to protect the health and wellbeing of both the participant him/herself, and of other participants in the study.

For trials that were begun before April 14, 2003, participants only need to sign an authorization form if reconsent is required. It should be noted that all PHI should be considered to be highly sensitive – however, if you follow principles of confidentiality then privacy in general should be maintained, regardless of the country you are practicing in.

EU Regulations

EU regulations are based on Directive 95/46/EC – also known as the Privacy Directive – which was enacted in 1995 and became law in the member states in 1998. The Privacy Directive covers all businesses that collect information, including, but not confined to, personal data that is collected during the course of a clinical research study.

Personally identifiable information is defined as: "any information relating to an identified or identifiable natural person ('data subject'); an identifiable person is one who can be identified, directly or indirectly, in particular by reference to an identification number or to one or more factors specific to his physical, physiological, mental, economic, cultural or social identity" [9].

This applies to all personal data collected during a clinical research study, but excludes data that have been "rendered anonymous in such a way that the data subject is no longer identifiable" [9].

Under the Directive, entities that collect information must tell the subject:

- who is collecting the information
- who will ultimately have access to it
- why the data is being collected

The subject also has the right to access and correct data about him/herself.

Applying Guidelines and Regulations

To ensure compliance with the guidelines and regulations that apply to your clinical research studies, you must ensure that you have a plan for how these will be implemented in practice. You are required to know the guidelines and regulations that apply to your research, but the next step in achieving responsible research is ensuring that your research is actually performed according to the rules. This can be achieved by training (you have a responsibility to make sure that both yourself and the rest of the research team are trained) and by SOPs (both by writing them and by ensuring that they are followed by the research team).

Training

With the introduction of new legislation to protect the privacy of individually identifiable PHI, clinical research professionals need to understand the obligations imposed by the applicable privacy legislation and the implications for their day-to-day practice.

As the CRC, you are designated the responsibility of implementing local country-specific privacy regulations regarding the PHI of individual subjects participating in clinical trials. This is true for all countries, including those that do not have privacy legislation in place, in which case you should follow the principles set out in ICH–GCP or in the "Declaration of Helsinki".

Training should not only focus on privacy issues, but should also cover GCP, especially as ICH–GCP states that everyone involved in a clinical research study should have the necessary skills to do their job effectively. Methods of training and learning are explored in more detail in **Chapter 12**, and it should be noted that you have a responsibility to ensure that the other team members are trained appropriately.

Standard Operating Procedures

The best way of ensuring that your research is conducted according to the rules and regulations is by having thorough SOPs. Indeed, ICH–GCP states that all parties involved in the conduct of clinical research, including sites, sponsors, and IRBs/IECs, should implement systems of procedures that assure the quality of every aspect of the trial; SOPs are very useful in this respect. **Table 6** provides the most important definitions relating to SOPs. A template SOP can be found in the **Appendix**.

SOPs allow guidelines and regulations for clinical research to be put into practice at a specific site, and you and the PI should follow these. Because SOPs act to ensure that GCP is followed and that the rights, safety, and wellbeing of clinical trial subjects are protected, you must play your part in the development, review, approval, and maintenance of SOPs at the site. Unfortunately, in reality CRCs often do not have as much time to spend on developing SOPs as they might like.

Development

In order for a clinical research site to be able to produce adequate SOPs, it must have a working group or committee that represents the research team, such as a formal clinical trials office with a quality assurance manager (or equivalent). If a site does

Term	Definition
SOPs	Detailed, written instructions that exist with the purpose of achieving the uniform performance of specific tasks
Compliance	The state of conforming with a legislative or regulatory requirement, or a recognized standard
Good Clinical Practice (International Conference on Harmonisation guidelines for Good Clinical Practice definition [2])	A standard for the design, conduct, performance, monitoring, auditing, recording, analysis, and reporting of clinical trials that provides assurance that the data and reported results are credible and accurate, and that the rights, integrity, and confidentiality of trial subjects are protected
Good Clinical Practice (Health Canada definition [10])	Generally accepted clinical practices that are designed to ensure the protection of the rights, safety, and wellbeing of clinical trial subjects and other persons, and the good clinical practices referred to in the definition for sponsor obligations in section C.05.010
SOP author	A member of the clinical research team or SOP committee qualified by experience, skills, and training to draft new or revised SOPs
SOP authorized signatory	An investigator or research team member qualified by experience, skills, and training to provide final approval of SOPs
SOP committee	A group of clinical research individuals responsible for the development, revision, review, and approval of SOPs. The committee should include a qualified investigator and a clinical research coordinator

Table 6. A summary of important terms related to standard operating procedures (SOPs) [2].

not have such a group then it must establish a formal SOP committee, which will be responsible for the continued review and approval process of SOPs at the site.

The role of the SOP committee is to establish formal processes for:

- the development, review, and approval of new SOPs
- the modification, review, and approval of currently used SOPs

It is essential that committee members remain aware of the latest changes to clinical trial guidelines and regulations in order to ensure that SOPs are created or updated as needed to reflect any changes to regulations, guidelines, research practice, or institutional policy.

The SOP committee should include an investigator and a CRC, and one member of the committee should be appointed as the SOP committee chair. The SOP committee should select someone who is qualified by experience, skills, and training to be the SOP author, who will draft new and revised SOPs – this is usually an experienced CRC or manager. This person should, of course, be familiar with the daily running of clinical trials at the site, but it is also important that he/she gets input from other members of the research team to obtain a group consensus.

It is important for a site to develop a process for SOP review and approval that works efficiently so that its SOPs are kept up-to-date. Draft SOPs should be circulated to the applicable reviewers (the SOP committee and other identified staff representatives) for comments. These comments should be incorporated and the revised draft SOP circulated to the SOP committee. The SOP committee will then review the final draft SOP for approval based on its accuracy and completeness, and its compliance with regulations, guidelines, and standard practice.

Review

The SOP committee should instigate a regular review process for all SOPs. SOPs should be reviewed at least annually – no later than 1 year after the effective date – as well as at any time that there are changes to regulations, guidelines, research practice, or institutional policies. If a site conducts early-phase clinical trials or trials involving high risks to subjects then SOPs should be reviewed more frequently, depending on the degree of risk. To ensure that timely updates occur, a review deadline should be set for each SOP.

When an SOP is reviewed, it needs to be assessed for:

- relevance
- practicality
- accuracy of content

There should also be a review of any attachments, along with any necessary updates to the SOP index. It is also important to analyze the methods used to conduct the SOP at the site: if the SOP is followed in different ways then it will need modifying. Some SOPs might need to be made more specific to the particular therapeutic areas of research or protocols conducted by a site. However, this does not mean that the SOPs will need to be modified for every protocol that the site works on; the SOP should cover all of the common ground for most types of protocols conducted by the site.

Central Files

Once an SOP has been reviewed, it is important for the SOP committee to complete an SOP review record and store it in a central SOP file. If a central SOP file does not already exist, the SOP committee should create one at the site, and only the SOP committee members should have access to it. The committee should be responsible for maintaining the central file and controlling access to the SOP documents.

A system for categorizing and numbering SOPs should be designed, as should a process for indexing and modifying different versions of SOPs and SOP templates. If paper SOPs are being used, SOP binders should be created and numbered, and a record kept of their location or the people to whom they have been distributed to ensure that all binders are updated simultaneously.

You should develop an SOP log and use this to document your SOP changes. Keep a record of the changes you make to SOPs and the reasons for the modifications. For example, if a new hospital policy dictates a change to a site's clinical research practice, the policy should be stated in the SOP or a reference made to the hospital policy. An SOP history template should be used as a chart to keep a record of any changes made to a site's SOPs. This can be stored in the central SOP file. All SOPs should be retained for 15–25 years from the effective date, depending on the requirements of your local authorities.

Documentation

As discussed previously, a site's SOPs need to be maintained and kept up-to-date. As well as making sure that clinical research is performed according to the guidelines and regulations, by keeping a record of reviews of and changes to SOPs the site will be ready for audits teams: the site will be required to show its procedures for conducting clinical research.

In addition, the process of following SOPs should help you to keep proper documentation of all the events involved in each clinical trial protocol – again, this will be needed for monitoring visits and site audits.

Communication

While the SOP committee's main job is to ensure that the site's SOPs are maintained and reflect the latest guidelines and regulations, it is all in vain unless the SOPs are readily available to all clinical research staff.

With paper SOPs, SOP binders should be made readily available to all clinical research staff at the site. All research staff must be notified of any changes made to the SOPs, and the rationale for the changes should be explained. The entire SOP document should be updated as necessary, including the overall table of contents section in the SOP binder. Additional attachments, such as required checklists or applicable regulatory documents, should also be included in the SOP binder.

For electronic SOPs, final SOPs should be posted in a format that cannot be altered (eg, as locked PDFs). Printed SOPs should be used as a reference only and destroyed after 14 days to ensure that the electronic files are checked regularly and only current SOPs are referenced.

As well as making new and revised SOPs available to staff, staff should also be trained on SOPs and/or a staff SOP review and sign-off policy should be implemented. All SOP training should be documented in the personnel records and a master list of training on each SOP should also be maintained in the SOP files.

Conclusion

The guidelines and regulations that you use to guide your clinical research practice are crucial. ICH–GCP is the worldwide standard for clinical practice and must be followed by all CRCs, in addition to recognizing the national regulations that apply to the country in which you are conducting research. Patient confidentiality and respect for privacy are also of vital importance, as you are the member of the research team who acts on behalf of the clinical trial participants.

It is not enough just to know the guidelines and regulations; the next step in achieving responsible research is ensuring that your research is actually performed according to the rules. This can be achieved by training and by creating SOPs. SOPs play a vital role in ensuring that research studies are performed in compliance with the guidelines and regulations; they act as a systematic set of procedures that ensure that the quality of every aspect of the study is maintained.

By being aware of the major guidelines and regulations, and by understanding how they should be implemented, you can ensure that your clinical research is safe and efficient.

References

1. Tri-Council Policy Statement: Ethical Conduct for Research Involving Humans 1998 (with 2000, 2002 updates). Medical Research Council of Canada; Natural Sciences and Engineering Council of Canada; Social Sciences and Humanities Research Council of Canada. Ottawa, ON: Public Works and Government Services Canada, 2003. Available from: pre.ethics.gc.ca/english/policystatement/policystatement.cfm. Accessed December 10, 2004.

2. International Conference on Harmonisation of Technical Requirements for Registration of Pharmaceuticals for Human Use. ICH Harmonised Tripartite Guideline: Guideline for Good Clinical Practice. E6. Available from: www.ich.org. Accessed November 17, 2004.

3. Juillet Y. The International Conference on Harmonisation of the Technical Requirements for the Registration of Pharmaceuticals for Human Use (ICH). Clinical Researcher 2002;2(12):28–35.

4. US Food and Drug Administration Code of Federal Regulations Title 21. Available from: www.accessdata.fda.gov/scripts/cdrh/cfdocs/cfcfr/CFRSearch.cfm. Accessed February 18, 2005.

5. NIH web site. Available from: www.nih.gov. Accessed February 18, 2005.

6. Canadian Institutes of Health Research, Personal Information Protection and Electronic Documents Act: Questions and Answers for Health Researchers. Ottawa, ON: Public Works and Government Services Canada, 2001.

7. Fedor CA. The coordinator's forum: follow-up to the effect of HIPAA. Clinical Researcher 2003;3(7):24–6.

8. Research Repositories, Databases, and the HIPAA Privacy Rule. NIH Publication Number 04-5489, 2004. Available from: privacyruleandresearch.nih.gov/pdf/research_repositories_final.pdf. Accessed February 18, 2005.

9. Directive 95/46/EC of the European Parliament and of the Council of 24 October 1995 on the protection of individuals with regard to the processing of personal data and on the free movement of such data. Available from: europa.eu.int/comm/internal_market/privacy/docs/95-46-ce/dir1995-46_part1_en.pdf. Accessed February 18, 2005.

10. Health Canada Therapeutic Products Directorate Food and Drug Regulations for Clinical Trials. Division 5. Canada Gazette Part II 2001;135(13): 1116–53. Available from: canadagazette.gc.ca/partII/tempPdf/g2-13513.pdf. Accessed February 18, 2005.

Chapter 3

Ethics and Human Subjects Protection

Felix A Khin-Maung-Gyi

Matthew Whalen

Introduction

Human subjects protection (HSP) spans issues such as consent (both the process of informed decision making and its documentation) and conflicts of interest, and is of great importance to clinical research coordinators (CRCs). While there are many facets to HSP, the issue of conflicts of interest has recently received the most attention, with one patient advocate organization even arguing that unless such conflicts are 'eradicated', the public should no longer volunteer for any clinical trials [1]. The current HSP climate would seem to be defined by a greater general awareness of the issues involved and their importance, and the realization that responsible, formal oversight is required to ensure that human research subjects are properly protected.

This added awareness, along with the increasing professionalism of clinical research, has resulted in voluntary certification programs for CRCs and monitors (also known as clinical research associates) and, more recently, a move towards the accreditation of entire clinical research institutions and organizations. In addition to the introduction of these voluntary standards, a new concept has been developed: that of human research protections programs (HRPPs). HRPPs are designed to ensure that all elements of a human research study – ie, staff, information systems, the research site, and all off-site partners/components – work together to protect the subjects of a trial. HRPPs will be discussed in more detail later in this chapter.

Mandatory standards also play a role in HSP; legislation regarding additional protections for research participants and the ethical conduct of research continues to be proposed in various national assemblies, and government oversight bodies across the globe are calling for more regulation and guidance. Of course, with increased responsibility comes a rise in litigation against those conducting and reviewing human research [2], accompanied by the specter of liability for those who fail to correctly interpret and follow the spirit of ethical research conduct and HSP regulations to the letter.

Therefore, for you, the professional CRC, heeding the adage 'good ethical research is good HSP' and paying close attention to compliance with HSP ethics and regulations is not an intellectual luxury, but a personal and professional obligation: a risk-management necessity, no less.

The Historical Context (1945–1999)

Consent

While the origins of what would, today, be recognized as clinical research involving humans can be traced back to 18th century Europe, the principle of obtaining 'voluntary consent' from those participating in clinical trials is inextricably linked to the first of 10 principles outlined in the "Nuremberg Code" [3]. This doctrine has been one of the foundations of the ethical conduct of research and of HSP. Recalling the horrifying experiments conducted on individuals in the concentration camps without their consent clearly puts the importance of this code into context as the primary tenet emerging from this tragic series of circumstances.

When considering the principle of voluntary consent, one of the most basic questions posed, both domestically and internationally, is: "Is it ethical to conduct research on a small number of people, with or without their consent and with or without personal benefit, if the results will benefit a larger number of people?" Clearly, there are divergent cultural responses. However, some societies' experiences, such as those of the USA, suggest that voluntary consent alone is not sufficient to assure the protection of human subjects.

The Birth of Ethical Oversight

In 1932, the US Public Health Service undertook an experiment to study the natural progression of untreated late-stage syphilis in Tuskegee, Alabama. In all,

Key events in the development of ethics and human subjects protection

The Hippocratic Oath
International ethical principles originated with the Hippocratic Oath, the earliest known code of medical ethics. The oath is attributed to Hippocrates, the 'father of medicine', who lived in the 5th century BC [11]. The oath is summarized as the principle of 'do no harm', and is the basis for the variety of oaths taken by most medical students in medical schools around the world.

The "Nuremberg Code"
In 1949, the "Nuremberg Code" - part of the official US report on the trials of Nazi war criminals after World War II - was published, becoming the first international code of ethics involving human subjects [3].

The "Declaration of Helsinki"
The "Declaration of Helsinki" is a globally recognized document that describes the standards for research involving humans [7]. It was established in 1964 and has been revised five times since, the last revision being in 2000. The declaration provides a comprehensive international statement on ethics and is the backbone for the International Conference on Harmonisation guidelines for Good Clinical Practice (ICH-GCP) [8].

The "Belmont Report"
The "Belmont Report" [5] is a US regulatory document that was drawn up in 1979 in response to an unethical study into syphilis. It defines three important ethical human rights: respect, beneficence, and justice. Also referred to as the Common Code, The "Belmont Report" embodies the fundamental ethical principles on which US federal legislation on clinical research is based.

600 men were studied between 1932 and 1972, including 201 'controls' (those without syphilis). The HSP problems were two-fold:

- Participants in the study were misinformed regarding the reasons for conducting the study.
- Appropriate medical care was withheld simply in the interest of understanding the natural progression of the disease.

Even though a treatment for syphilis had been discovered and was widely available during the 1940s, the study continued as planned causing needless suffering for the rural, poor, African–American men who were enrolled. After the study came to the public's attention via the news media and an associated series of governmental hearings were convened, ethical principles were developed to govern research. These principles resulted in the "Belmont Report" and regulations mandating the involvement in, and oversight of, research by a review committee. These principles still form the backbone of current regulations.

This review committee is what is now referred to in the USA as an institutional review board (IRB) or, internationally, as an independent ethics committee (IEC), ethics review committee, or ethics review board, which by title reinforces the ethical dimension of research review deliberations. It is the duty of these bodies to assure the protection of the rights and welfare of research participants.

In the context of US research, the word 'institutional' in IRB needs to be put into perspective. Historically, the models under which research has been conducted have consisted primarily of academic medical centers and teaching hospitals. It was accepted and understood that the 'institution' was where research would be conducted, and so centralized yet independent oversight within the institution was deemed sufficient.

Conflicts of Interest

Today's clinical research environment is highly competitive, both in terms of the business aspect and of recruiting research subjects, so traditional perceptions of how clinical research should be structured and HSP provided have proven to be inadequate. HSP must span not only concerns of voluntary consent and physical and psychological harm, but also potential (real or perceived) harm from pressures resulting from researchers' and sponsors' financial and nonfinancial conflicts of interest.

A recent US example of a tragedy associated with conflicts of interest and HSP was the death of an 18-year-old research participant in a gene therapy trial. In 1999, the young man enrolled in a nontherapeutic study designed to determine the effects of administering an adenovirus vector. However, following participation he died secondary to hematologic complications. The principal investigator was an equity owner in the company developing the product, as was the University of Pennsylvania, where the study was approved and conducted. The prevailing theory is that the investigator's objectivity as a scientist and clinician was clouded by his desire to gain academic recognition and benefit from the resulting financial interests.

Compliance and Conscience

At around the time of the gene therapy trial tragedy and the legal wrangling over conflicts of interest, several highly regarded academic medical centers and government-supported healthcare institutions in the USA were subject to regulatory scrutiny, criticism, and, in some cases, shutdown due to poor (or a complete lack of) compliance with clinical research regulations. Examples of noncompliance included, among others, a lack of essential administrative processes – eg, documentation of meeting minutes – and a failure to follow appropriate procedures at convened meetings.

In the case of the University of Pennsylvania and, more recently, the Johns Hopkins Medical Institutions, the circumvention of regulatory processes and procedures resulted in the death of research participants. To borrow useful phrases from Dr Greg Koski, the first Director of the Office of Human Research Protections (OHRP) of the US Department of Health and Human Services, these tragic and unacceptable outcomes appear to reflect the institutions' failure to adopt a "culture of conscience", let alone a "culture of compliance".

Similarly, institutional directives that appear to tolerate questionable intent, whether consciously or not, can add to the perception that HSP is not held in high esteem within an organization. In the past 3 years in particular, many have argued that HRPPs should be accredited, so that objective or defined standards of conduct can be used to measure an organization's compliance with both regulatory guidelines and ethical principles. In these circumstances it will soon be possible to find out, both in the USA and internationally, whether there is any truth behind the maxim 'morality and ethics cannot be regulated'. Standards and acceptability criteria will have to be defined for ethics-based practices, and this must be done in the context of global medical research.

The Five Ethical Principles

Using ethical principles, one could take a supporting or opposing point of view on any given topic and argue that position effectively. In clinical research, the coexistence of the cultures of compliance and conscience poses a particular challenge. When faced with ethical dilemmas, one needs to be heroic in taking a stand by exercising moral courage.

A Canadian attorney/ethicist has provided a succinct perspective: "The science–spirit view recognizes that there is more that we can do with our new science than what we ought to do... This view requires the courage to live with the uncertainty that making… [ethical] distinctions involves" [4]. Here is our challenge: to apply moral courage in the clinical research setting. How we do so involves the application of ethical principles to our daily research work.

To draw from the seminal 1979 US regulatory document the "Belmont Report", three principles can be identified [5]. It is important to note that the "Belmont Report" was drafted in response to events that resulted from the exposure of the Tuskegee Syphilis Study. It is also worth noting that, of all US federal regulations, Good Clinical Practice regulations are the only ones that are actually founded on ethical principles. The core ethical principles articulated in the "Belmont Report" are:

- respect for persons
- beneficence
- justice

To these three it is useful, practically speaking, to add:

- permission
- compassion

Respect for Persons

The Belmont principle of respect for persons is about taking into account the individuality of subjects and not just seeing them as members of a group or class, and also respecting individuals and their right to choose to participate in research. Simply put, it is the application of the first principle of the "Nuremberg Code" – voluntary consent. In addition to obtaining informed consent, 'respect' implies and assumes that protections will be provided for those who could be exploited, whether their vulnerability is social, economic, educational, or related to gender, race, age, or anything else.

Beneficence

The Belmont principle of beneficence can be summarized as 'do to others their good' or 'minimize harm while maximizing benefits'. In this construct, beneficence goes beyond the medical dictum 'do no harm'; 'good' expands to embrace psychological, social, and economic benefits, and more.

Justice

The Belmont principle of justice can be succinctly described as 'equitable benefits for equitable risks'. The notion of distributive justice reminds us to be fair in our imposition of risks to individuals, particularly regarding who receives the benefits and bears the burdens of research. Those who benefit from the research should be those who bear the risks. In other words, a vulnerable group should not be exposed to research from which they will not benefit.

Permission

The principle of permission is, "Do not do to others that which they would not have done unto them, and do for them that which one has contracted to do" [6]. Here, permission is really the principle of informed decision making, and includes contracts – written and verbal – and all that they imply. (See **Chapter 5** for more on the informed consent process.)

Compassion

As a principle, compassion is the foundation of the other principles, emphasizing that ethics is fundamentally an interactive reality. That is, ethical principles involve a self engaging and interacting with other(s) where 'enlightened self-interest' is achieved through achieving the interests of others.

Research versus Practice

One of the single biggest issues in international research (especially in developing and redeveloping countries) is the blurring of the distinction between research and practice – for all too many, research becomes healthcare. The ethical issue here is that the focus of the research becomes treatment versus data, which leads to research subjects misunderstanding the intent of the research. This, in turn, leads to a lack of understanding (an issue of consent).

Part A of the "Belmont Report" helpfully differentiates between clinical research and clinical practice, and provides additional guidance when discerning whether certain activities are research or not. The key differences between research and practice are listed in **Table 1**.

Data derived from research help to establish appropriate treatment guidelines, which can be applied daily in evidence-based medical practice. Similarly, using

Practice	Research
• Purpose is to provide diagnosis, preventive treatment, or therapy to particular individuals • Interventions are designed solely to enhance the wellbeing of an individual patient/client, which should have a reasonable expectation of success	• An activity designed to test a hypothesis, permit conclusions to be drawn, and to develop or contribute to generalizable knowledge • Usually described in a formal protocol that sets out an objective and a set of procedures designed to reach that objective

Table 1. The differences between medical practice and research.

good clinical research practice helps those involved to identify reasonable hypotheses from which to derive additional research. As professionals, we have adopted the notion of practicing evidence-based medicine. We have now reached a point where we need to practice principle-based research in order to:

- sustain the clinical research enterprise
- re-establish 'trust' in this enterprise
- assure the acceptability and integrity of data
- simply, 'do the right thing'

Historical experiences such as Nuremberg and Tuskegee remind us that simply pursuing good science will not result in ethical research. As the field of clinical research continues to expand and become more complex, infusing a culture of conscience into the entire research process – from developing ethical research protocols to retention of study subjects – becomes a practical necessity. In order to answer scientific questions, good HSP is good clinical research, which, in turn, is the application of good ethical behavior.

The Ethical Challenges Facing CRCs

In general, what are called 'ethical' issues are frequently not; rather, many issues are clinical, legal, regulatory, social/public policy, and/or administrative. It is important to discriminate between these, because identifying an issue as one of ethics can potentially impact its discussion in negative ways:

- unnecessary levels of uncertainty can be introduced
- the diversity of opinion can be increased

Part A of the "Belmont Report"

It is important to distinguish between biomedical and behavioral research on the one hand, and the practice of accepted therapy on the other, in order to know what activities ought to undergo review for the protection of human subjects of research. The distinction between research and practice is blurred partly because both often occur together (as in research designed to evaluate a therapy) and partly because notable departures from standard practice are often called 'experimental' when the terms 'experimental' and 'research' are not carefully defined.

For the most part, the term 'practice' refers to interventions that are designed solely to enhance the wellbeing of an individual patient or client and that have a reasonable expectation of success. The purpose of medical or behavioral practice is to provide diagnosis, preventive treatment, or therapy to particular individuals. By contrast, the term 'research' designates an activity designed to test an hypothesis, permit conclusions to be drawn, and thereby to develop or contribute to generalizable knowledge (expressed, for example, in theories, principles, and statements of relationships). Research is usually described in a formal protocol that sets forth an objective and a set of procedures designed to reach that objective.

When a clinician departs in a significant way from standard or accepted practice, the innovation does not, in and of itself, constitute research. The fact that a procedure is 'experimental', in the sense of new, untested, or different, does not automatically place it in the category of research. Radically new procedures of this description should, however, be made the object of formal research at an early stage in order to determine whether they are safe and effective. Thus, it is the responsibility of medical practice committees, for example, to insist that a major innovation be incorporated into a formal research project.

Research and practice may be carried on together when research is designed to evaluate the safety and efficacy of a therapy. This need not cause any confusion regarding whether or not the activity requires review; the general rule is that if there is any element of research in an activity, that activity should undergo review for the protection of human subjects.

These factors can both make a discussion (such as an IRB/IEC deliberation) or a decision needlessly complex or sensitive. For example, at a site going through an audit or an IRB/IEC accreditation process, the majority of issues raised are related to (usually a lack of) documentation of activities defined in standard operating procedures rather than ethics. While inadequate procedures might suggest an inattention to the ethical conduct of research, they are not in, and of, themselves necessarily indicative of overt violations of ethical principles.

There are two dimensions to ethical behavior:

- a person's role and responsibilities
- the interaction of that person's role with others and their responsibilities

Put differently, ethical conflicts can arise by a person either not fulfilling their role or failing to interact responsibly with others. This is a particularly important frame of reference for HRPPs (see the discussion later in this chapter, p. 46).

Professional and national governmental mandates do indeed have an ethical impulse and are frequently founded on ethical principles. Such mandates span the US Code of Federal Regulations and guidance provided by the "Declaration of Helsinki" [7], the International Conference on Harmonisation [8], and the Council for International Organizations of Medical Sciences (through individual medical codes of conduct) [9]. However, the crucial part is the interpretation of mandates at the level of day-to-day experience. Specific examples of the kinds of ethical challenges you might face will now be discussed using the five principles stated earlier.

Respect for Persons (Autonomy)

Research participants interact with CRCs personally, directly, and intimately, so this is perhaps the most accessible and understandable principle under your direct control. Examples of situations in which a CRC may intentionally or unintentionally affect an individual's autonomy when making a decision to participate in research include:

- providing misleading information to potential participants that might bias their decision to enter a study
- offering financial or nonfinancial (such as emotional) inducements that might influence a potential participant's decision to participate in research
- using spoken and/or nonverbal communication that might influence a potential participant's independence

All instances of coercion (or use of unduly influencing tactics such as monetary incentives) fall into this category. Respect for persons also includes other ethical and clinical responsibilities to the research participant, especially with regards to populations who might be considered 'vulnerable' and who should be afforded additional protections.

Definitions of 'vulnerability' can depend on multiple factors, and can include the indication being studied in addition to the participants themselves. In relation to clinical issues, the application of this principle includes adequate and appropriate medical oversight of research participants during and following research. Some sources, such as the recent revisions to the "Declaration of Helsinki" in 2000 and 2002, suggest that the sponsors of research should continue to provide medication to research participants even after completion of the study, if clinically appropriate.

Beneficence (Maximize Benefits and Minimize Risks)

While those responsible for designing the way in which the research will be conducted are best equipped to maximize the application of this principle, there are also multiple opportunities for you to apply this principle in both clinical and nonclinical settings. As the CRC, you are in a good position to provide feedback to the sponsor on the real-world feasibility of a study, such as the personal impact of the study on a volunteer – eg, about procedures that might cause loss of wages or even jeopardize employment due to absenteeism.

Very importantly, you can also fulfill this ethical principle by submitting reports of serious and unanticipated adverse events in a timely fashion to both the sponsor of the research and the overseeing IRB/IEC, and by keeping abreast of what, if any, additional risks have arisen to subjects as a result.

Justice (Fair Selection of Subjects)

Matters of injustice that you might come across include:

- conducting a study whose results cannot possibly benefit the subject population and the subject's community or family
- enrolling a 'professional subject' whose recent involvement in another clinical trial (typically a Phase I study) jeopardizes the cleanliness of the data, and hence impacts upon the safety of future users of the investigational drug/device.

Permission

Examples of challenges involving the principle of permission include:

- performing procedures not required in the protocol
- suggesting benefits of participation to potential subjects that are not supported by the study
- changing the way that informed consent is taken by shortening the IRB/IEC-approved consent form without seeking new IRB/IEC approval, even if it appears to make the form more understandable

- failing to give potential subjects adequate time to consider whether to participate

It is worthwhile noting that breaches of privacy can also fall under violation of the principle of permission.

Compassion

Finally, compassion – a fundamental principle of ethics in both western and eastern traditions – can affect CRCs in particularly profound ways. It can be argued that conflicts of interest – financial and otherwise – violate the principle of compassion, allowing the interests of the study and/or the study staff to supersede the interests of the subject.

Perhaps most significantly, compassion is a matter of personal character that can guide your professional conduct as a whole, as it can the study designer, the investigator, and the IRB/IEC member, among so many others in clinical research.

Human Research Protections Programs (HRPPs)

HRPPs are most closely identified with IRB/IEC accreditation, but are more than that. While accreditation is ideally geared to go beyond formal regulations, laws, and guidance as the foundation of HSP – by promoting best practices and continuous process improvement – it is not the apex of HRPPs. Indeed, in order to go beyond a culture of compliance and toward a culture of conscience, an HRPP is a more thorough system that ties together various constituents of the clinical research enterprise both internally (ie, within an organization, whether a freestanding site or a major medical center) and externally (eg, between an organization and the trial sponsor or the IRB/IEC). To illustrate this, an HRPP within a healthcare facility encompasses not only the clinical research professionals conducting the research, but also the education programs that support them, the IRB/IEC, and the administrative functions – from leadership to information systems – that interact with the clinical research effort. **Figures 1** and **2** illustrate HRPPs from both the internal and external perspectives, and are extensions of the proposals of Dr Greg Koski, the first Director of the OHRP.

The ties that bind HRPPs together might be legal contracts or defined communications channels. Regardless of these ties, the system is one of mutual assurances, reinforced by the encouragement of, and actual support for, ethical

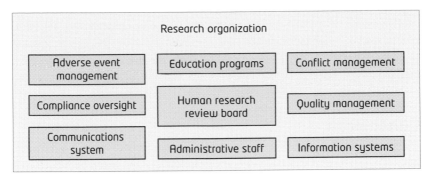

Figure 1. Human research protections programs: internal elements of an effective program. Adapted from Dr Greg Koski, ACRP presentation, Toronto, Canada 2002.

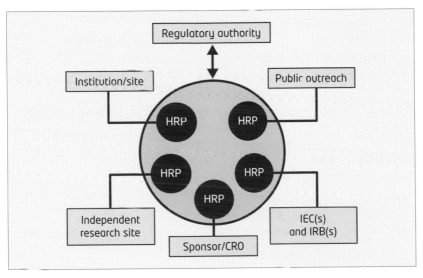

Figure 2. Human research protections programs: an external viewpoint. CRO: contract research organization; HRP: human research protections; IEC: independent ethics committee; IRB: institutional review board.

judgments in the form of investments in clinical research activities. Such investments range from fiscal to physical (space, equipment); from intellectual (dedicated expertise) to human resource capital (staff support).

Taken in their most meaningful way, HRPPs are codified by site accreditation and the certification of clinical research professionals, and they also embody the culture of conscience. HRPPs are intended to increase domestic and international public confidence in, and understanding of, the clinical research enterprise. As such, HRPPs go far beyond documentation and the letter of the law; they are the guiding spirit of HSP and actively, and continually, apply the five core ethical principles outlined in this chapter.

Conclusion

Ethics is no longer a privileged domain isolated from the real world of clinical research. There are three key messages you should remember:

- In our industry, making good ethical decisions and good business decisions can be one and the same thing.
- Making good decisions is, in no small part, a matter of applying the five guiding principles in the course of decision making.
- A 'culture of conscience' goes beyond sheer compliance and is a matter of individual self-development efforts that involve, first and foremost, personal change in order to lead cultural change.

References

1. Harvard Partners. Almost 1/2 of faculty on IRBs have ties to industry. New York (NY): Alliance for Human Research Protection; 2003, August 15. Available from: www.ahrp.org/infomail/ 03/08/15.php. Accessed November 17, 2004.

2. Mello MM, Studdert DM, Brennan TA. The rise of litigation in human subjects research. Ann Intern Med 2003;139:40-5.

3. The Nuremberg Code. In: Trials of War Criminals before the Nuremberg Military Tribunals under Control Council Law No. 10. Washington, DC: US Government Printing Office, 1949;2:181-2. Available from: ohsr.od.nih.gov/guidelines/nuremberg.html. Accessed November 17, 2004.

4. Somerville MA. The Ethical Canary: Science, Society, and the Human Spirit. Toronto, Ont: Viking/Penguin Canada, 2000:20-1.

5. National Commission for the Protection of Human Subjects of Biomedical and Behavioral Research. Belmont Report: Ethical Principles and Guidelines for the Protection of Human Subjects of Research. Washington, DC: US Government Printing Office, 1979.6. Engelhardt HT, Jr. The Foundation of Bioethics, 2nd edn. New York, NY: Oxford University Press, 1996:123-4.

7. The World Medical Association. World Medical Association Declaration of Helsinki. Ethical Principles for Medical Research Involving Human Subjects. Available from: www.wma.net/e/policy/b3.htm. Accessed November 17, 2004.

8. International Conference on Harmonisation of Technical Requirements for Registration of Pharmaceuticals for Human Use. ICH Harmonised Tripartite Guideline: Guideline for Good Clinical Practice. E6. Available from: www.ich.org. Accessed November 17, 2004.

9. Council for International Organizations of Medical Sciences. International Guidelines for Biomedical Research Involving Human Subjects. Geneva: CIOMS, 2002. Available from: www.cioms.ch/frame_guidelines_nov_2002.htm. Accessed November 17, 2004.

10. The World Medical Association. World Medical Association Declaration on the Rights of the Patient. Available from: www.wma.net/e/policy/l4.htm. Accessed November 17, 2004.

11. Jones WHS, translator. Hippocrates. Cambridge, MA: Harvard University Press, 1923:289.

Chapter 4

Responsible Conduct of Research

Philip A Cola

Eric M Cottington

Introduction

During the past 15 years, integrity in research and academic scholarship has come to be commonly described as the "responsible conduct of research". However, this term is not necessarily recognized or fully understood by many people involved in clinical research – including clinical research coordinators (CRCs) – so an improved understanding of what is involved would be extremely beneficial to the clinical research enterprise.

According to the US Department of Health and Human Services Office of Research Integrity (ORI), the topics most often covered in discussions of responsible conduct of research include [1]:

- conflicts of interest
- mentoring
- authorship and publication
- data management
- ethics and morality
- research misconduct
- human subjects protection (HSP)

As ethics, morality, and HSP are covered in **Chapter 3** of this handbook, this chapter will focus on the other areas. A general overview of conflicts of interest in research will be given (see **Chapter 3** for further information on the effects of conflicts of interest on HSP), along with a discussion of mentoring, authorship and publication, data management, and research misconduct. This will act as an introduction to these issues, to help you to become more aware of them and to feel more comfortable with addressing them in your day-to-day experiences.

Conflicts of Interest in Research: a General Overview

It is important for you to understand the definition and scope of conflicts of interest in research. Conflicts of interest often derive from investigators' personal and financial interests in clinical research, as well as their intellectual endeavors. These biases might influence investigators and affect the interpretation of published research data, which can eventually lead to mistakes in clinical practice [2]. It is necessary to identify and manage these biases in order to maintain the public's trust in clinical research.

It is critical to review and understand potential conflicts of interest in the early stages of the research process, not only to ensure research objectivity, but also as their identification and management could significantly affect HSP [3].

Financial Conflicts of Interest

From your perspective, the most common or readily identifiable conflicts of interest will be financial. Financial conflicts of interest occur when there is a perception that investigators or research staff stand to gain financially from the results of the research, when these individuals are responsible for the design, conduct, or reporting of the research.

Although financial gains can exist, they need to be managed when certain monetary thresholds are reached. Examples of financial conflicts of interest according to the US Public Health Service (PHS) include [4,5]:

- salary or payments for services, such as consulting fees or honoraria, which are expected to exceed US$10,000 in a 12-month aggregate period for individuals or their immediate families

- equity interests, such as stock options, with a fair market value over US$10,000 or that represent more than a 5% ownership in any single entity for individuals or their immediate families
- intellectual property rights such as patents, copyrights, and royalties from the rights

You need to be aware of these commonly accepted concepts and definitions in order to recognize and assist in the management of financial conflicts of interest.

Currently, financial conflicts of interest are receiving increased attention because of a growth in research funded by private industry, interest in technology transfer activities in academic medical centers, and publicity surrounding perceived abuses at research institutions [6–8]. The effects of financial conflicts of interest on research may be significant and include [9]:

- issues relating to the publication of results that favor a sponsor's product
- a lower scientific validity of the research
- subjection of the data to prepublication review or restrictions
- a lower likelihood that researchers will disseminate the results to the entire scientific community

Managing Conflicts of Interest

Conflicts of interest occur in all types of research. However, conflicts of interest in research involving human subjects must be treated differently compared with basic research. HSP rules and regulations require, though not explicitly, that investigators and CRCs fully inform potential participants of any potential conflicts that might affect an individual's decision to participate in the research [10]. You must recognize that the extent of disclosure and the prohibitions regarding financial interests should be greater when doing human subject research.

Institutional review boards often require conflicts of interest to be disclosed, so that they can deliberate on the issues and make recommendations to ensure the protection of the human subjects participating in the research. As the fundamental contact for study subjects, you will be responsible for managing the full disclosure of any potential issues during the informed consent process and subsequent study visits. Therefore, you need to understand your institution's policies relating to conflicts of interest and be familiar with your institution's integrity guidelines on this topic.

Strategy	Explanation
Public disclosure	Informing institutions, IRB, staff, the community, and study participants that there is a conflict
Additional monitoring or oversight of research	Having independent investigators obtain consent, conduct study visits, and/or analyze and report data
	More frequent IRB review
Divestiture/prohibition of financial interests	Eliminate all conflicts before commencing with the research
Disqualification from/ discontinuation of research	Find new investigators or institutions to conduct the research
Modification of research design	Change the study population, outcome measures, data safety monitoring functions, and data analysis to limit the effect of the conflict
Refusal of funding	Not allowing financial gain
Placing equity in escrow	Delaying financial gain
Donating proceeds from equity to other organizations	Not allowing direct financial gain

Table 1. Strategies for managing conflict of interest. IRB: institutional review board.

Institutional policies on conflicts of interest vary widely [8,11]. You can help to monitor disclosure and to ensure full disclosure to appropriate institutional officials or committees on issues that arise or those that are perceived as potential conflicts. Ultimately, these committees will recommend a strategy for managing the conflict and you must understand what this strategy will entail when overseeing the day-to-day conduct of a clinical research study. A list of strategies often used to manage conflicts of interest is given in **Table 1**.

Both you and the principal investigator (PI) must be aware of your ability to appeal a committee's recommendations regarding a conflict of interest decision, and you must also understand that there will be sanctions for investigative teams who do not comply with institutional policies.

Mentoring

Developing expertise as a mentor requires time and experience, regardless of the role you play in conducting research. Therefore, it is vital that new members of the team conduct research studies alongside seasoned veterans before taking on independent roles and responsibilities. Investigators must also be aware that they will need mentoring themselves – usually by senior investigators, but sometimes by officials at the institution where they are conducting the clinical research.

At times, however, it can be easy to forget or ignore fundamental duties relating to the responsibility for education and training. The pressure to enroll study subjects can, alone, interfere with the need to take time out for mentoring duties. More often, responsibilities such as overseeing the conduct of a study, the informed consent process, study enrollment, data analysis, and the publication of results overshadow the importance of mentoring and training study staff. Therefore, being aware of the responsibilities that mentorship brings will enable you to focus on fulfilling them. After all, good mentoring is just as important as normal study duties for ensuring the responsible conduct of research.

Teamwork and Communication

Mentorship is important in helping study team members to understand their roles. Mentors must recognize that clinical research is impossible unless strong, productive team relationships are established. Investigators cannot conduct clinical research without you, and you cannot conduct clinical research without investigators and other team members. Responsible research requires investigators to delegate to experienced and qualified individuals such as CRCs, and CRCs must also be able to delegate some of their duties to other qualified members of the team.

Investigators should seek advice from experienced investigators and embrace the fact that they have overall responsibility for the conduct of the study. As the CRC, you should recognize that you are responsible for the day-to-day conduct of a study, and you should update investigators in an efficient manner, as well as sharing what you have learned with the rest of the study team. Administrative assistants, data managers, recruitment specialists, and others will look to you for advice on their role in a study and, if you are an experienced CRC, it is likely that the PI will direct you to provide mentorship for them.

However, CRCs often take on many studies and within any given study you might take on many different roles [12]. This, along with the high workload of many investigators in fast-paced academic medical centers or private practices, prohibits the level of interaction that is necessary to build a strong mentor–trainee relationship. Therefore, you will need to play an active role in the mentor–trainee relationship and consult with the investigator to help clearly define the roles of the other team members. This is an educational process similar to informing a potential study subject of his/her role as a participant in a research study.

You need to be sure that you understand the protocol completely and you should recognize that the best way to ensure complete understanding is to discuss any issues with the investigator or study sponsor. Understanding the institutional HSP program and knowing who to seek advice from about the conduct of research are also important. The utilization of excellent communication skills is vital to successful mentorship, and you must be able to discuss sensitive issues in a constructive manner. Communication is discussed further in **Chapter 11**.

Training and Education

A good mentor will know the importance of training and education. Because guidelines and regulations dictate that investigators must be adequately trained and show core competencies in human subjects research, most academic institutions have created formal clinical research education and training programs. It is critical to take advantage of the training opportunities offered by institutions and sponsors, and to know who to ask to gain information in a timely manner.

There are often financial implications of training and education, with institutional and departmental budgets often only allowing for limited training and educational resources. The sponsor's study budget usually allows for some level of training for study investigators and their staff, so good negotiating skills are vital to secure the appropriate funds.

Knowing which of these training opportunities will cater to your specific needs at a given time in your career development will allow for the efficient use of the available educational resources. All research team members must create time for formal learning or training activities in their otherwise busy schedules. Investigators must be willing to make time to participate in and attend educational seminars provided by institutions and research sponsors, and should also allow time for (and encourage) CRCs to attend such programs. These opportunities might come before or after regular work hours, but are important to pursue in order to ensure that research is conducted in a responsible way. **Chapter 12** discusses learning in greater detail.

Authorship and Publication

As the CRC's role in conducting clinical research continues to grow, the topic of authorship, in relation to the publication of the results of research, is becoming more relevant for CRCs. According to the US National Institutes of Health (NIH), authorship is "the fulfillment of the responsibility to communicate research results to the scientific community for external evaluation." It is also "the primary mechanism for determining the allocation of credit for scientific advances, and thus the primary basis for assessing a scientist's contributions to developing new knowledge" [13].

Because of the importance of authorship, principles of responsible authorship have been developed. These principles are meant to guide individuals and groups when making decisions regarding who should be included as an author on a paper. For example, the authorship requirements identified by Wilson are outlined in **Table 2** [14].

In addition to following these principles and guidelines with respect to defining authorship, there are also factors to consider when determining who the primary (or first) author should be. Houk and Thacker state that the primary author should contribute one or more of the following [16]:

- originality of the contribution (ie, he/she has developed a novel idea or research question to pursue)
- the major intellectual input
- the major feature of the manuscript
- the greatest overall contribution

It is very important that the members of the research team understand and agree to these principles of authorship at the outset of the project, especially for clinical research projects, which typically involve teams. You must be able to discuss issues of authorship with the PI as a project commences; disputes often arise later about who should be included as an author, or the order in which the authors should be listed. Such disputes can be contentious and difficult to resolve, and it is best to avoid or minimize them by agreeing these matters in advance. The principles described above can help guide these efforts.

- Authors must have participated sufficiently in the work so as to take public responsibility for its content.
- Authors must be willing to respond to questions about the work.
- Authors must make substantial contributions to all of the following (from 'the uniform requirements for manuscripts submitted to biomedical journals' [15]):
  - conception and design, or acquisition of data, or analysis and interpretation of data
  - drafting the article or revising it critically
  - final approval of the version to be published
- The following are not sufficient to justify authorship:
  - participating solely in the acquisition of funding
  - participating solely in the collection of data
  - supervising the overall activities of the research group

Table 2. The requirements for authorship, as identified by Wilson [14].

Data Management

Data management is a critical factor in the success of any research project. According to the NIH, "research data, including detailed experimental protocols, all primary data, and the procedures of reduction and analysis, are the essential components of scientific progress" [13]. To this end, one needs to understand three key concepts:

1. what research data are
2. why data management is so important
3. what the critical areas of data management are

What are Research Data?

There is little consensus on the definition of research data; the definition can vary according to the discipline or the sponsor of the research. While bench scientists may view research data as experimental observations recorded in laboratory notebooks (eg, of cells grown in culture) or electronic data from scientific instruments, behavioral scientists may view research data as audio or video recordings of behavior, or questionnaires received from subjects. **Table 3** outlines the definitions of 'data' in use by several organizations.

Part of the US Food and Drug Administration's definition (ie, data that are "necessary for the reconstruction and evaluation" of a report of the research) is a common feature of most definitions of research data used by research universities and professional organizations. In addition, many organizations stress the

Organization	Notes and definition
Federal Acquisition Regulations	Govern most federal research contracts
	Define data as: "recorded information, regardless of form or the media on which it may be recorded" [17]
Public Health Service	No formal definition of research data
Food and Drug Administration	Defines research data in part of its Good Laboratory Practice for Nonclinical Laboratory Studies as: "Laboratory worksheets, records, memoranda, notes, or exact copies thereof, that are the result of original observations and activities of a nonclinical laboratory study and are necessary for the reconstruction and evaluation of the report of that study. In the event that exact transcripts of raw data have been prepared (eg, tapes which have been transcribed verbatim, dated, and verified accurate by signature), the exact copy or exact transcript may be substituted for the original source as raw data. Raw data may include photographs, microfilm or microfiche copies, computer printouts, magnetic media, including dictated observations, and recorded data from automated instruments" [18].

Table 3. Definitions of data.

importance of primary data, that is, the original (source) data rather than compiled or derived data. In the clinical research arena, where industry sponsorship is common, the research data is captured on individual subject case report forms, with primary data emanating from source documents such as patient medical records.

Why is Data Management Important?

There are four main reasons for being concerned about how research data are managed:

1. research integrity
2. intellectual property protection
3. ensuring confidentiality
4. compliance with the sponsor's requirements

Research Integrity

Research integrity requires "the meticulous attention to the acquisition and maintenance of data" [13]. Sloppy science, and sloppy data management practices in particular, can lead to questions about the validity of the findings. Inspecting and reanalyzing the research data often answers these questions, but if the primary data are not available or are of questionable quality then integrity is compromised. You must understand that data from clinical trials are monitored to gather additional safety information (ie, adverse events and unanticipated problems) as well as to ensure the integrity of the compiled data [19].

Intellectual Property Protection

According to the NIH, research data are legal documents for purposes of establishing patent rights [13]. Legal challenges to ownership often require production of the original data, complete with dates. Therefore, attention to good data management practices will help to ensure the protection of intellectual property. You will often be at the forefront of the data collection process, and so you need to be aware of general data ownership issues.

Ensuring Confidentiality

Sponsors and institutions might want data to be kept confidential for proprietary or security reasons, eg, until a patent can be filed to protect intellectual property. In addition, HSP regulations might require data to be kept confidential.

This requirement has become more prominent with the implementation of the Health Insurance Portability and Accountability Act in the USA, the Personal Information Protection and Electronic Documents Act in Canada, and Directive 95/46/EC (the Privacy Directive) in the EU, which exist to protect the privacy of personal health information. In summary, concerns about confidentiality will dictate how data is collected, retained, and shared.

Compliance with the Sponsor's Requirements

As part of a grant or contract, sponsors will often have specific requirements regarding how long data should be kept, with whom data can be shared, and who has rights to the data. For example, many sponsors (eg, the NIH) require all data to be kept for a period of 3 years following the submission of the final financial report.

Industry sponsors will be concerned about who has rights to the data. Industry sponsors usually own the rights to de-linked case report form data, and research institutions usually maintain ownership of and protective responsibilities for the source documentation. It is important for investigators and CRCs to read and understand the sponsor's terms and conditions regarding data as they relate to a grant or contract, and to work with institutions to negotiate changes where necessary.

What are the Critical Areas of Data Management?

There are four main data management practices that deserve careful attention:

1. data acquisition
2. data analysis
3. data sharing
4. data retention

Data Acquisition

The NIH has noted that research data should be carefully recorded in a form that will allow continuous access for analysis and review [13]. Lack of attention to proper data acquisition practices (eg, inaccurate or biased recordings, and/or incomplete records) can clearly affect the integrity of research and the ability to defend its integrity. The interim monitoring of data is required on a regular basis [19].

Data Analysis

Data analysis is also of concern with respect to research integrity. The US National Academy of Sciences has stated that "It is a violation of the most fundamental aspect of the scientific process to set forth measurements that have not, in fact, been performed (fabrication) or to ignore or change relevant data that contradict the reported findings (falsification)" [20]. For example, the exclusion of data from an analysis on the basis of them being 'outliers' is problematic and, generally, should be avoided.

Data Sharing

The general norms of science emphasize the principles of openness. To this end, members of the academic community will often freely share data, including research materials, with colleagues and collaborators. This practice can conflict with the expectations of industry sponsors in particular, who often view data as proprietary. Also, patient privacy concerns might limit the extent of data sharing that is allowed.

Data Retention

The directives for data retention given by the International Conference on Harmonisation guidelines for Good Clinical Practice are outlined in **Table 4** [21].

"**4.9.5** Essential documents should be retained until at least 2 years after the last approval of a marketing application in an ICH region and until there are no pending or contemplated marketing applications in an ICH region or at least 2 years have elapsed since the formal discontinuation of clinical development of the investigational product. These documents should be retained for a longer period however if required by the applicable regulatory requirements or by an agreement with the sponsor. It is the responsibility of the sponsor to inform the investigator/institution as to when these documents no longer need to be retained."

Table 4. The International Conference on Harmonisation (ICH) guidelines for Good Clinical Practice - directives for data retention [21].

These require the retention of essential documents for at least 2 years. Some sponsors, however, specifically require that data be kept for a period of 3 years following the completion of a research project, and there can even be a requirement for longer retention periods. This might be necessary in order to have the original data to defend challenges to the integrity of the research, or to protect the intellectual property resulting from the research.

For example, some institutions require that research data be retained for a period of 3 years or until the publication of the research, whichever is longer. Industry sponsors might require that the data be retained for a period of 3 years from marketing approval of an investigational drug or device. You will play a crucial rule in understanding and disseminating information regarding data management to the other research team members.

Research Misconduct

Historically, universities had research misconduct offices that investigators in the university might have been aware of; however, CRCs in affiliated hospitals did not necessarily know where or to who misconduct should be reported [22]. The main emphases when discussing the responsible conduct of research are generally best practices or model behaviors. However, concerns about misconduct in research, which came to light in the 1980s, have caused federal agencies and institutions to generate policies that specifically define and address behaviors that constitute research misconduct.

Most policies define these behaviors as plagiarism, fabrication, or falsification in proposing, performing, or reviewing research, or in reporting research results.

> **Plagiarism** is the appropriation of another person's ideas, processes, results, or words without giving appropriate credit.
>
> **Fabrication** is making up data or results and recording or reporting them.
>
> **Falsification** is manipulating research materials, equipment, or processes, or changing or omitting data or results such that the research is not accurately represented in the research record.

Table 5. Behaviors that constitute research misconduct, as presented in the April 2004 proposed rule for the US Public Health Service [23].

The PHS also includes in its definition of research misconduct the following phrase: "other practices that seriously deviate from those that are commonly accepted within the scientific community for proposing, conducting, or reporting research" [23]. A proposal to eliminate this phrase from the PHS definition has been communicated to the scientific community and may be adopted in the near future. All definitions of research misconduct exclude "honest error or honest differences in interpretations or judgments of data" [1].

A more detailed description of the behaviors that constitute research misconduct is outlined in **Table 5**.

Reasons for Misconduct

Misconduct can result from various influences. Certainly the pressure to publish or obtain research funding in order to be promoted or receive tenure at an academic institution can cause some individuals to engage in research misconduct. CRCs might feel pressured to enroll subjects or to produce results in order to ensure enough grant funding exists to maintain their current employment status. However, conflicts of interest and personality differences among colleagues, or conflicts between faculty and students, can also lead to misconduct situations. False allegations of misconduct can also be made to retaliate against perceived unfair treatment.

Because allegations of research misconduct can have a devastating effect on the careers of the individuals involved, it is important for an institution to have a clear, well organized set of procedures for responding to such allegations.

Procedures for Dealing with Misconduct

Most institutions' procedures for dealing with allegations of research misconduct are based on the recommendations of the ORI. Institutions generally follow specific steps when responding to an allegation of misconduct. These steps include:

- an inquiry phase
- an investigation phase
- a report
- appeals

An institutional official (eg, a research integrity officer) is usually identified as being responsible for hearing allegations, and for deciding whether an allegation is credible and meets the definition of research misconduct. An allegation can be either in writing or given orally. If the research integrity officer determines that an allegation is credible and meets the definition of research misconduct then an inquiry panel (usually composed of the researcher's peers) is formed. This panel collects additional information, generally though interviewing the person bringing forth the allegation and reviewing other pertinent information, such as original research records.

If the inquiry panel believes that the evidence is sufficient to warrant an investigation then the research integrity officer forms an investigation panel (again, usually composed of the researcher's peers) and a formal investigation is initiated. This investigation involves more interviews with key individuals and the careful review of original research records and related material. Generally, a preponderance of evidence is required to substantiate an allegation of research misconduct.

The investigation panel prepares a report of its findings, which is shared with both the person making the allegation and the person about whom the allegation is made. Comments are solicited and a final report is compiled, including a recommendation and sanctions, as applicable. This report is generally sent to an institutional 'deciding official', who is not the research integrity officer. This person makes the final decision as to whether the investigation panel's recommendation should be accepted or rejected. This final decision is then reported to the various parties and sometimes to the sponsoring agency, as required by appropriate regulations. The person about whom the allegations have been made can then make an appeal.

Key factors in effectively addressing research misconduct at an institution include:

- clear, well-communicated policies and procedures
- a responsible research integrity officer to administer the policy
- peers who are willing to serve on inquiry and investigation panels

- a timely process (it is important to have deadlines by which to complete each phase of the process)
- the ability to maintain confidentiality (for all involved) and to sequester original research records as necessary

A major task for you will be to engage investigators to take responsibility when misconduct issues are raised about other CRCs, investigators, or even the PI him/herself. You must cultivate a relationship in which issues relating to misconduct can be appropriately and openly discussed. Too often, CRCs are uncomfortable with such issues, but you need to know that a compliance office exists that can assist with these complicated situations [22].

Conclusion

It is critical for you to understand the areas of responsible conduct of research that are covered in this chapter in order for you to conduct clinical research appropriately. You need to be able to recognize conflicts of interest and/or issues of data management/integrity when they arise. Even areas that have not historically been commonly addressed by CRCs in their day-to-day activities (ie, the management of conflicts of interest, authorship, etc) are important for you to understand and to confront as necessary.

References

1. Steneck NH. Introduction to the Responsible Conduct of Research. Rockville, MD: US Department of Health and Human Services, Office of Research Integrity, 2004.

2. Korenman SG, Shipp AC. Teaching the Responsible Conduct of Research Through a Case Study Approach: A Handbook for Instructors. Washington, DC: Association of American Medical Colleges, 1994.

3. Martin JB, Kasper DL. In whose best interest? Breaching the academic-industrial wall (Erratum appears in N Engl J Med 2001;344:536). N Engl J Med 2000;343:1646–9.

4. Federman DD, Hanna KE, Rodriguez LL, editors. Responsible Research: A Systems Approach to Protecting Research Participants. Washington, DC: National Academies Press, 2002.

5. Title 42, US Code of Federal Regulations, Part 50.601. Available from: www.gpoaccess.gov/cfr. Accessed December 6, 2004.

6. National Science Foundation. Investigator financial disclosure policy. Fed Reg 1995;60:35820-3.

7. Angell M. Is academic medicine for sale? N Engl J Med 2000;342:1516-18.

8. Morin K, Rakatansky H, Riddick FA Jr, et al. Managing conflicts of interest in the conduct of clinical trials. JAMA 2002;287:78-84.

9. Lo B, Wolf LE, Berkeley A. Conflict-of-interest policies for investigators in clinical trials. N Engl J Med 2000;343:1616-20.

10. Barnes M, Krauss S. Conflicts of interest in human research: risks and pitfalls of "easy money" in research funding. Health Law Reporter 2000;9:1378-86.

11. Siang S. Money talks: financial conflicts of interest. Clinical Researcher 2000;1(0):34-7.

12. Fedor C, Cola P. The Coordinators' Forum. Preliminary results of the Clinical Researcher coordinators' survey. Clinical Researcher 2003;3(4):18-22.

13. Guidelines for the Conduct of Research in the Intramural Research Programs at NIH. Available from: www.nih.gov/campus/irnews/guidelines.htm. Accessed December 6, 2004.

14. Wilson JR. Responsible authorship and peer review. Sci Eng Ethics 2002;8:155-74.

15. International Committee of Medical Journal Editors. Uniform requirements for manuscripts submitted to biomedical journals. JAMA 1997;277:927-34.

16. Houk VN, Thacker SB. The responsibilities of authorship. In: Editorial Policy Committee of the Council of Biology Editors, editors. Ethics and Policy in Scientific Publication. Bethesda, MD: Council of Biology Editors, 1990:181-4.

17. Title 48, US Code of Federal Regulations, Part 27.401. Available from: www.arnet.gov/far/current/html/Subpart_27_4.html. Accessed December 6, 2004.

18. Title 21, US Code of Federal Regulations, Part 58. Available from: www.cfsan.fda.gov/~lrd/cfr583.html. Accessed January 21, 2005.

19. Slutsky AS, Lavery JV. Data safety and monitoring boards. N Engl J Med 2004;350:1143-7.

20. National Academy of Sciences. Responsible Science: Ensuring the Integrity of the Research Process, Vol. 1. Washington, DC: National Academy Press, 1992:47.

21. International Conference on Harmonisation of Technical Requirements for Registration of Pharmaceuticals for Human Use. ICH Harmonised Tripartite Guideline: Guideline for Good Clinical Practice. E6. Available from: www.ich.org. Accessed January 21, 2005.

22. Cola P. Definition of scientific misconduct requires accurate interpretation and enforcement. Clinical Researcher 2002;2(9):26-9.

23. Department of Health and Human Services. Public Health Service policies on research misconduct. Proposed rule. Fed Reg 2004;69:20777-803.

Chapter 5

The Informed Consent Process

Philip A Cola

Why is Informed Consent Important?

The most critical aspect of conducting ethical clinical research is the process of obtaining informed consent from study participants [1,2]. In research, informed consent refers to the study participant's prospective agreement to participate in a research study once he/she has gathered enough essential information to independently make that decision [2]. The need to obtain voluntary informed consent from human subjects participating in research was the first, and main, principle that emanated from the "Nuremberg Code", which was drawn up after the Nuremberg war crimes trials [3].

When discussing informed consent, it is essential to appreciate that it is not a single event or merely a form to be signed, but rather the core educational process that takes place between the investigators, study staff, and prospective participants. It is also important for all parties to understand that the process continues for the duration of the research, since the participant can withdraw his/her consent at any time without prejudice, and information might accrue that will affect the willingness of the participant to continue in the study.

Even though the process is aimed at the study participant and, ultimately, it is the responsibility of the investigator, as the clinical research coordinator (CRC) you are the key research team member in the informed consent process. In order to appropriately conduct the informed consent process, you will often assume the role of participant advocate. Additionally, you will be intimately involved with all aspects (scientific, ethical, and practical) of the study. This makes you the person

• An explanation of the purpose of the study and that it is a research project (ie, describe what is being studied and why)	• A description of the possible risks involved and any discomfort that might occur
• An explanation of why the potential study participant is being asked to participate (eg, because he/she is a normal volunteer, has a particular condition, or meets certain other criteria)	• A description of the possible benefits
	• Disclosure of the alternatives to participation
	• Assurances of confidentiality
	• An explanation of the concept of the voluntary nature of participation
• A full explanation of the study procedures that will be followed, including:	• An explanation that the participant has the right to refuse to participate and to withdraw without penalty
– the duration of participation (the number and length of visits and follow-up visits)	• Disclosure of any costs and compensation related to participation
– the study design (whether the trial involves drug-free periods, randomization, blinding, and/or placebo control; whether it is researching efficacy, safety, or tolerability; what phase the study is; what groups of subjects are participating; and what investigational treatments or procedures will take place)	• Contact information for research team members who can answer participants' questions, and be contacted in the event of an adverse event or injury
– a discussion of research versus standard care (if applicable)	

Table 1. Elements of the informed consent document.

who is most knowledgeable about all aspects of the study, in addition to being the person who is most accessible to the participant.

Worldwide, informed consent must be obtained prospectively from the participant or his/her legally authorized representative (in the USA, some details might differ slightly according to individual state laws relating to issues such as surrogate consent). It cannot be obtained after screening or after the initiation of study procedures, nor can it be obtained through a third party, unless the study calls for the inclusion of special populations (discussed later in this chapter) and the local jurisdiction legally allows for such variation in this process.

The participant must have the cognitive and psychological capacity to understand the information being conveyed to him/her or special procedures and safeguards

- Title 45 CFR Part 46.111 (a)(4) requires adequate comprehension on the part of the subject
- Title 45 CFR Part 46.116 (8) specifies the voluntary choice to participate
- Title 45 CFR Part 46.116 (1) states a requirement for full disclosure of the nature of the research and the participant's involvement

Table 2. US regulations specifying the three essential elements of informed consent.

must be introduced into the process to help ensure understanding, such as additional assessments, special review bodies, or the involvement of family and friends. These special procedures and safeguards accentuate existing approaches, but become even more relevant in special populations.

The Informed Consent Document

The physical informed consent document must contain a minimum of eight basic elements of informed consent, as required by federal regulations in the USA (Title 45 Code of Federal Regulations [CFR] Part 46.116 and Title 21 CFR Part 50.25) and by the International Conference on Harmonisation guidelines for Good Clinical Practice (ICH–GCP) throughout the world, including the EU, Japan, and Canada [4]. A more complete listing of each element of informed consent is provided in **Table 1** [2,4,5]. Three of the essential elements are:

- adequate comprehension on the part of the subject
- the voluntary choice to participate
- full disclosure of the nature of the research and the participant's involvement

Table 2 lists the US regulations that specify these three essential elements. In recent years, some research professionals have suggested that these elements, which are used by investigators and CRCs to discuss and obtain informed consent, essentially become the subject's 'bill of rights' for participating in clinical research [6]. The use of this terminology accentuates the importance of these elements and they may also be referred to as 'human subject rights' [7].

- Use simple language and a large font size
- Make documents shorter and the text less dense
- Summarize information in tables
- Use section headings to break-up the text
- Embolden text to emphasize key points
- Provide an outline or a table of contents
- Provide a glossary
- Leave space in which questions can be written during the informed consent process

Table 3. Strategies by which to communicate complex informed consent concepts.

Ensuring Understanding

Ensuring Understanding During the Informed Consent Process

The informed consent process must begin with [8]:

- an understandable explanation of the research procedures
- a clear statement that the intervention is research and that the encounter and study-related procedures to be followed are related to research
- a clear statement that research is the "dissemination of generalizable knowledge"

These, and all other elements of study participation, must be described in lay language at approximately an eighth-grade (13 years of age) reading level for adults in the USA and other developed countries, and at a third- to fifth-grade (8–10 years of age) reading level in special study populations or developing countries.

In order to bridge the gap between complex issues and terms and the ability of the participant to understand the information, you will become an interpreter. You must work closely with institutional review boards (IRBs)/independent ethics committees (IECs) and sponsors to find the most effective approaches to communication. **Table 3** provides some examples of ways in which complex concepts can be communicated to participants in an informed consent document.

Readability of the Informed Consent Document

Historically, concerns have been raised about the process of informed consent because it is an inexact science. More recently, these concerns have grown because consent forms have continued to increase in complexity and the methods employed to communicate information to diverse audiences of adults and children are not consistently adequate [9]. Many recent studies have indicated innovative ways to improve the informed consent document – through attention to readability standards, use of an easy-to-read layout, and use of audiovisual presentations or graphical summaries – with the ultimate goal of increasing potential participants' understanding of and confidence in the study [9–12].

It would seem straightforward to follow these recommendations and to simplify consent forms by using the suggested methods. However, the legal language recommended by study sponsors, institutions, and sometimes even IRB/IEC members often complicates the ability to simplify written documents to levels that would be more understandable [13]. Study sponsors might desire the language to be taken verbatim from the federal regulations as they fear litigation [9].

The additional consent language required by these groups can result in consent forms that contain more information than is actually required, and the language can seem to be aimed at satisfying the sponsor's or institution's needs rather than those of the study participant [13]. You play a critical role in balancing the sponsor's and institution's requirements with the need to simplify the informed consent document; you must do this without delaying the conduct of the study while ensuring that, ultimately, study participants will understand the final consent document.

Reviewing the Requirements of Participation
The next step is to review all of the requirements of participation with the potential participant; this includes a very detailed discussion and description of each procedure called for by the research protocol. It is critical for the risks and benefits of participation to be presented in the informed consent process, and participants will require an assessment of the risk to benefit ratio of the study to make an informed decision about participation [14].

You must also review the frequency of contact with the participant and the duration of participation, including an explanation of the number of visits required, the assessments that will take place at each visit, and the length of time that the visits are expected to last. It is also common to discuss travel to and from the study site and the personal needs (ie, time away from work, child care, family involvement,

Aspects of participation to be reviewed with the participant:
- procedures
- risks and benefits
- frequency of contact
- duration of participation visits: assessments and length
- travel
- participant's personal needs
- the purpose of the study

Table 4. Informed consent discussion checklist.

meals, etc.) of the participant. A checklist for the informed consent discussion is provided in **Table 4**.

After these temporal requirements and inconveniences have been covered in detail, it is always useful to re-emphasize the purpose of the research study and why the potential participant is being approached for participation.

Assessing Comprehension

Measures of comprehension must be both valid and reliable [15]. Many attempts at assessing comprehension fail to take both of these variables into consideration. The assessment of comprehension of the informed consent document is an area that is critical to your role. In order to measure comprehension appropriately, you must have:

- clinical expertise in the area particular to the research study
- a sound methodology to employ when attempting to measure this important aspect of the informed consent process

There is a paucity of good research data on the use of various comprehension tools, or methods, to gauge understanding of informed consent in clinical research. Often, supposed tools are crude and not proven to be reliable in the area of measuring comprehension. For example, neuroscience investigators might propose to use a tool such as the brief psychiatric rating scale or the mini mental state examination to gauge a potential participant's ability to comprehend information.

Recent strategies that have been employed to test comprehension include a series of true–false questions, paraphrasing documents in writing [15], or a test/re-test approach through a series of questions (verbal and/or written) to see if participants are generally grasping the information provided as well as measuring the amount of information retained. Currently, there are no globally accepted standards for measuring comprehension of the informed consent document, and so you, the CRC, become even more important in your attempts to ensure participant comprehension. Often, you must rely on clinical skills and follow-up questions that will help you to establish the level of the participant's understanding.

Obtaining Informed Consent

Requirements for Obtaining Consent

It is not just CRCs who are involved in the informed consent process. Principal investigators, co-investigators, research assistants, and other research team members (with sufficient knowledge of the research protocol and responsible conduct of research) can, with the appropriate training and ample time, also obtain informed consent from participants.

In the USA, research professionals obtaining informed consent must be trained in the areas of human subjects protection (see **Chapter 3**) and responsible conduct of research, as required by federal, local, and institutional standards [5]. Such standards for training now also exist in Canada, but are currently less formalized in Europe and Japan. In Japan, the Ministry of Health and Welfare does require general training for CRCs relating to research conduct, but this differs to the specific human subjects protection training that is required in the USA. These training requirements improve the standard of human subjects protection and help to increase recruitment rates, while ensuring that appropriate participants are enrolled (this also improves participant retention).

Participants must have ample time in which to make informed decisions about enrolling in a clinical trial. Time must be allotted for the participant to ask questions and involve others, as required, in order to make an informed decision. Rushing through the process because of time-related constraints on you or the investigator could potentially be harmful to the participant. You should consider keeping track of the amount of time it takes to complete the initial and subsequent informed consent processes for a given study, and use this data as a benchmark to compare subsequent participant enrollment, and enrollment into similar studies [16].

Building Relationships with Participants

You will find yourself in a special, trustworthy position with potential study participants, and will serve a primary role as advocate. One of the major reasons why people enroll and remain in a study is the relationship that they develop with the CRC during the informed consent process [14]. Physicians can sometimes influence or intimidate participants, especially when the physician is both the investigator and the participant's treating physician. You, however, will often be seen as a neutral party who will take the time to discuss important issues or questions with participants.

Your ability to simplify complex information into lay language will also help to build a strong, trusting relationship with study participants. When a study requires multiple visits, these relationships will become more important because you will be spending a good deal of time with the study participant throughout the completion of the research protocol. You will become the main constant at the site for the participant, and you will be the person who has 'all the answers', while still taking the time to respect any concerns that the participant may have. In the case where you are also the subject recruiter, the participant will have an even stronger identification with you, as you will have been their constant point of contact from prestudy discussions through to visits during the study.

Interpersonal Skills

During the informed consent process, you must present the basic required elements of informed consent to the potential study participant and make every effort to ensure that he/she adequately comprehends the information. To be able to do this properly, you must understand the study thoroughly. During this initial phase of the consent process, a bond will begin to develop between you and the potential participant; the participant will be relying on you to convey information in a simplified and relaxed manner, and you will be getting to know the potential participant and understand his/her motivation for taking part in the study.

Although sponsors, investigators, and IRBs/IECs all expend energy ensuring that consent forms are written in a way that is easy to understand, it is you who will be faced with ensuring that the study information is conveyed in a way that maximizes comprehension. You must be able to further simplify the explanation of complex research procedures, the concept of research versus routine medical treatment, and risk to benefit ratios.

Reviewing Key Issues with the Participant

Avoiding Undue Influence and Misconceptions

It is very important for consent to be given without coercion or undue influence. You must build a level of trust with participants and ensure that you do not coerce them in any fashion when they are making decisions. You must speak and interact with each participant at the appropriate level; this is often very individual to the participant and not necessarily to the study. It is critical for the study subject population to be identified appropriately, and not merely for the convenience of you or the investigator. This is the basic ethical principle of justice (see **Chapter 3** for further discussion) as it relates to study participant recruitment [8,17], and it will help you to avoid potentially exerting undue pressure or influence.

Once any potential study team influences have been removed, external misconceptions and myths must be dealt with. A common problem occurs when a patient with a particular medical condition becomes a potential study participant, and is inadvertently misled by the hope for improved treatment of their affliction. This is a common misunderstanding and is referred to as the 'therapeutic misconception' [5,18].

Another problem can arise from the fact that individuals usually have an inherent trust in what they believe a physician or healthcare professional is recommending to them. Therefore, physicians and CRCs who are involved in the informed consent process must be very careful to not unduly persuade people into participating in research. It must become standard practice for ongoing communication regarding the rights and welfare of study participants to take place throughout the study. Participants must not, in any manner, be made to give up any of their legal rights or be given the impression that they are being asked to do so [19].

Participants Can Say "No"

Once the concepts behind the research have been explained and understood, a discussion of the voluntary nature of participation should follow. It should be made clear to the participant that they have a choice about whether or not to participate in the research, and that there are usually other treatment options available to them outside of the clinical trial. The participant's power to say "no" to participation is fundamental to the concept of true informed consent and to the right to withdraw at any time without prejudice.

Other Aspects Required for Proper Informed Consent

Time and the Physical Environment

The manner and context in which information is conveyed is as important as the information itself. The research team members involved in informed consent must be willing to assign adequate time for the process to be completed comfortably. Participants should not be rushed through the informed consent process because of a research professional's busy schedule. It takes time to explain the concept of research to individuals who are not accustomed to the practice of research by their everyday lives.

Study procedures are often complex for individuals outside of the healthcare profession, even for those who are well educated, so during the process it is mandatory to provide the chance for questions to be asked and satisfactory answers received. Because investigators cannot always commit enough time to the informed consent process, the task is usually delegated to CRCs, who are often already experienced at working closely with potential participants.

Due to the nature of the personal interaction between you and the participant, the physical environment of the study site and the personality and communication skills of the CRC are key variables that can impact on the success of subject enrollment into clinical research studies.

Documentation of Consent

In the USA, the process of obtaining informed consent must comply at all times with the requirements of Title 45 CFR Part 46.116 and Title 21 CFR Part 50.20. Informed consent must be documented by investigators and CRCs in compliance with Title 45 CFR Part 46.117 [19,20], and participants must be comfortable with the process.

Universally, the study sponsor will monitor these requirements throughout the study and will require that the consent process is documented in the research records (ie, source documents and case report forms) to the level of including written statements about what was done during the process of informed consent, who participated in the informed consent process, and the date and time at which the consent process took place.

The Ongoing Process of Informed Consent

After the physical form has been signed, the process of informed consent is ongoing throughout the study [19]. If new information arises during the course of the study then participants need to be informed of this information so that they can have the opportunity to decide whether to continue participating or to exercise their right to withdraw from the study. It is possible that new information will change the risk to benefit ratio, especially if the information is related to the safety or efficacy of the treatment under investigation. You must be able to recognize this potential change, and you should inform the IRB/IEC in order to seek advice about the level and depth to which the currently enrolled participants should be updated, as well as strategies for informing new participants through the informed consent process.

It is vital to re-establish the consent process throughout the research protocol (ie, at each visit an interaction regarding ongoing understanding must take place between you and the participant). In the case of progressive cognitive disease, or for other special study populations, it is essential to reconfirm; this confirmation should be documented each time it occurs.

Research in Special Populations

Obtaining Informed Consent

Special populations participating in research require particular provisions during the informed consent process. Examples of special research populations include pregnant women, individuals with temporarily or permanently impaired decision-making ability, institutionalized people (eg, prisoners, hospitalized patients, or long-term care-facility residents), students, institutional employees, and participants who are considered minors as defined by local laws.

Such populations must have research studies made available to them, as excluding them from the opportunity to participate in research would violate the ethical principle of justice [17], as well as giving the perception that their issues somehow warrant less consideration than others [21]. To appropriately include such special populations in research studies, you need to be aware of these special populations and to understand the regulations and guidelines that apply to them.

Regulations and Guidelines

US regulations for including pregnant women, prisoners, and children in research are clearly outlined in 45 CFR 46, Subparts B, C, and D, respectively (pediatric assent is examined further in **Chapter 6**) [20]. Many other countries do not have formal regulations specifically addressing these populations. However, the EU has a general "Pediatric Rule" and Australia has also developed guidance on pediatric research. CRCs around the world must be familiar with these various regulations prior to participating in the informed consent process with these populations.

However, a greater challenge for you will be understanding the various guidances and suggestions regarding the inclusion in research of participants with temporarily or permanently impaired decision-making ability. This latter group includes, for example, people with Alzheimer's disease, schizophrenia, or other major mental disorders, and stroke patients. There are no consensus regulations on the inclusion of these populations in research, so you must understand local laws and institutional policies and recognize the tools available to you for including these subjects appropriately in research. When attempting to enroll people from these populations, it is necessary for you to obtain additional information before, during, and after the informed consent process.

Currently, there are no regulations anywhere in the world that specifically govern the inclusion of decisionally impaired participants. However, in the USA guidelines have been issued in an attempt to ensure additional protections [22]. These guidelines allow for additional assessments, special reviews, and the involvement of family or friends of the participant in the informed consent process, and also remind investigators and CRCs to carefully consider the need for the specific study population while minimizing risks and maximizing benefits. This information can include [23]:

- ratings of the individual's ability to understand the information being presented to him/her
- the ability to utilize proxy, surrogate, or advanced consent
- ongoing assessment of the participant's ability to understand the research study

Conclusion

Your challenge is to make the informed consent process as effective as possible, which will, ultimately, result in greater protection for human subject participants in research. You serve a fundamental role in the informed consent process and must remember that conducting research with human participants is ultimately a privilege granted by willing volunteers and not merely a transaction to meet study enrollment quotas [24].

References

1. Rosse PA, Krebs LU. The nurse's role in the informed consent process. Semin Oncol Nurs 1999;15(2):116-23.

2. Ethics and research. In: Burns N, Grove SK, editors. The Practice of Nursing Research: Conduct, Critique, and Utilization. 4th ed. Philadelphia, PA: WB Saunders Company, 2001:191-222.

3. The Nuremberg Code. In: Trials of War Criminals before the Nuremberg Military Tribunals under Control Council Law No. 10, Nuremberg, October 1946-April 1949. Washington, DC: US Government Printing Office, 1949,?:181 2. Available from: ohsr.od.nih.gov/guidelines/nuremberg.html. Accessed November 17, 2004.

4. International Conference on Harmonisation of Technical Requirements for Registration of Pharmaceuticals for Human Use. ICH Harmonised Tripartite Guideline: Guideline for Good Clinical Practice. E6. Available from: www.ich.org. Accessed November 17, 2004.

5. Federman DD, Hanna KE, Rodriguez LL, editors. Responsible Research: A Systems Approach to Protecting Research Participants. Washington, DC: National Academies Press, 2003.

6. Getz K, Borfitz D. Informed Consent: The Consumer's Guide to the Risks and Benefits of Volunteering for Clinical Trials. Boston, MA: CenterWatch, Inc., 2002.

7. Hochhauser M. Improving patients' understanding of research: A plain English summary and informed consent form. Clinical Researcher 2003;3(12):16-27.

8. McGuire Dunn C, Chadwick G. Protecting Study Volunteers in Research: A Manual for Investigative Sites. Boston, MA: CenterWatch, Inc., 1999.

9. Palladino ML. Challenges in the informed consent process: identifying design strategies that enhance communication in adult clinical trials. Research Practitioner 2002;3(5):164-71.

10. Paasche-Orlow MK, Taylor HA, Brancati FL. Readability standards for informed-consent forms as compared with actual readability. N Engl J Med 2003;348(8):721-6.

11. Shea K. Visual design in the informed consent process. Research Practitioner 2002;3(5):172-4.

12. Schapira MM, Meade C, Nattinger HB. Enhanced decision-making: the use of videotaped decision-aid for patients with prostate cancer. Patient Educ Couns 1997;30(2):119-27.

13. Ruth K. IRBs contribute to consent form complexity. Clinical Researcher 2003;3(3):6-7 (News item).

14. Ginsberg D. The Investigator's Guide to Clinical Research. 2nd ed. Boston, MA: CenterWatch, Inc., 1999.

15. Hochhauser M. Informed consent: Reading and understanding are not the same. Applied Clinical Trials 2004;April:42-48.

16. Sharp SM. Common problems with informed consent in clinical trials. Research Practitioner 2004;5(4):133-7.

17. National Commission for the Protection of Human Subjects of Biomedical and Behavioral Research. Belmont Report: Ethical principles and guidelines for the protection of human subjects of research. Washington, DC: US Government Printing Office, 1979.

18. Appelbaum PS, Lidz CW, Grisso T. Therapeutic misconception in clinical research: frequency and risk factors. IRB: Ethics & Human Research 2004;26(2):1-8.

19. Office for Protection from Research Risks. Tips on informed consent. Revised March 16, 1993. Available from : www.hhs.gov/ohrp/humansubjects/guidance/ictips.htm. Accessed January 18, 2005.

20. US Food and Drug Administration Code of Federal Regulations Title 45, Part 46, Subparts B, C, and D. Available from: ohsr.od.nih.gov/guidelines/45cfr46.html. Accessed January 18, 2005.

21. Dresser R. Mentally disabled research subjects. The enduring policy issues. JAMA 1996:276(1):67-72.

22. National Bioethics Advisory Commission. Research Involving Persons with Mental Disorders That May Affect Decisionmaking Capacity. Volume 1. Rockville, MD: US Government Printing Office, 1998. Available from: www.georgetown.edu/research/nrcbl/nbac/capacity/TOC.htm. Accessed January 18, 2005.

23. Karlawish JH, Knopman D, Clark CC, et al. Informed consent for Alzheimer's disease clinical trials: a survey of clinical investigators. IRB: Ethics & Human Research 2002;24(5):1-5.

24. Ramsay MAE. Responsible research: the clinical trials office. Clinical Researcher 2002;2(11):4-5.

Chapter 6

Pediatric Informed Consent and Assent

Barbara J Daly

Introduction

Research using children as subjects presents several kinds of challenges, both to those involved in the conduct of research and to those charged with overseeing and protecting the rights of children. Since the publication of the "Belmont Report", there have been specific norms, rules, and provisions in regulations intended to ensure that children are adequately protected [1]. Research with children requires investigators to address two major questions, both stemming from the limitations in decision-making capacity that are typically found in children. It is well accepted that persons who possess full decision-making capacity are in the best position to make judgments about the degree of risk to which it is reasonable to expose themselves, or the amount of burden associated with participation that is acceptable. Clearly, in general, children do not have the same ability to make these judgments and to protect themselves.

Thus, as a society we believe that we should in some way limit what is done to children, regardless of, or in addition to, any consideration of who can give consent or permission.

The rules promulgated by the US Department of Health and Human Services (HHS) in Title 45 Code of Federal Regulations Part 46 (45 CFR 46) – "Protection of Human Subjects" – include specific sections that impose limits on the acceptable research risks to children, and outline the requirement that the child's wishes be given weight regarding participation [2]. The US Food and Drug Administration (FDA) also imposes rules governing research and has adopted most of the requirements of 45 CFR 46 [3]. Similar regulatory requirements exist in many European countries [4,5].

In addition to limiting what research can be done, we also have the same moral obligation to demonstrate respect for children as we do for adults [6]. Recognition of this obligation requires us to create ways to inform potential child research-subjects about proposed research participation and to seek their agreement or disagreement. This is a complex challenge for many reasons, and it requires careful planning and implementation of consent procedures by research staff.

This chapter provides an overview of the current regulations governing the inclusion of children in research, particularly in relation to the requirements for parental permission and child assent. Guidelines for the process of obtaining permission and assent will also be discussed.

Sources of Guidance

Historical Developments

The first widely accepted rule regarding research ethics, the "Nuremberg Code", was interpreted as prohibiting the participation of children as research subjects. The first principle of the code states, "The voluntary consent of the human subject is absolutely essential" [7]. Thus, children were excluded because they lack decisional capacity.

It was not until the "Belmont Report", which was drafted in 1979 by the National Commission for the Protection of Human Subjects of Biomedical and Behavioral Research, that it was recognized that there was a need for specific guidelines for persons who were impaired either in their cognitive capacity or in their ability to give truly voluntary consent [1].

The "Belmont Report" was prompted by the recognition that the general standards outlined in the "Nuremberg Code", for use with the Nuremberg trials of war criminals, were insufficient to address the complex situations arising in contemporary research. The National Commission recognized that:

- The capacity for decision-making is not absolute, but rather exists on a continuum.

- The protections of persons in the context of research should be relative to their ability to make their own decisions and to the risks and benefits of the proposed research.

The report further recognized that the principle of justice demands that classes or groups of people ought not to be excluded from the potential benefits of research, but that the characteristics of groups that might make them vulnerable to harms must be considered when selecting subjects and designing relevant protections.

Since the issuance of the "Belmont Report", US regulations governing the conduct of research with humans have attempted to address both the need to include children in research, and the need for specific guidelines to regulate when children may serve as subjects and how to protect their rights.

Over time, as funding agencies have established policies requiring children to be included in research unless there are sound reasons to exclude them, 45 CFR 46 has been updated repeatedly to expand on the special considerations for pediatric research subjects (subpart D) [2]. In addition, the FDA has recognized the need to adequately test and label drugs for use in pediatric populations. In 2001, the FDA modified its regulations – 21 CFR 50 and 21 CFR 56 – to adopt essentially all of the provisions of 45 CFR 46, subpart D [3].

A similar evolution in regulatory oversight has occurred in other nations. By 1990, the International Conference on Harmonisation (ICH) had been formed by regulatory authorities in the EU, Japan, and the USA. The purpose of this multinational coalition is to make recommendations on ways to promote greater consistency in research guidelines and the requirements for pharmaceutical approvals. Both the ICH and the UK Medical Research Council have identified minors as a vulnerable population that warrants extra protection in research [4,5]. The EU Clinical Trials Directive also offers guidance on clinical trials on minors (see **Table 1**) [8].

Current Regulations
The federal regulations applicable to pediatric research have two major aspects:

- rules relating to the conditions under which children may be included in research
- rules relating to authorization from either legally recognized proxies (usually parents) or children themselves

- The informed consent of the parents or legal representative has been obtained; consent must represent the minor's presumed will and may be revoked at any time, without detriment to the minor.
- The minor has received information according to its capacity of understanding, from staff with experience with minors, regarding the trial, the risks and the benefits.
- The explicit wish of a minor who is capable of forming an opinion and assessing this information to refuse participation or to be withdrawn from the clinical trial at any time is considered by the investigator or where appropriate the principal investigator.
- No incentives or financial inducements are given except compensation.
- Some direct benefit for the group of patients is obtained from the clinical trial and only where such research is essential to validate data obtained in clinical trials on persons able to give informed consent or by other research methods; additionally, such research should either relate directly to a clinical condition from which the minor concerned suffers or be of such a nature that it can only be carried out on minors.
- The corresponding scientific guidelines of the Agency have been followed.
- Clinical trials have been designed to minimise pain, discomfort, fear and any other foreseeable risk in relation to the disease and developmental stage; both the risk threshold and the degree of distress have to be specially defined and constantly monitored.
- The Ethics Committee, with paediatric expertise or after taking advice in clinical, ethical and psychosocial problems in the field of paediatrics, has endorsed the protocol.
- The interests of the patient always prevail over those of science and society.

Table 1. Conditions under which clincal trials on minors can be undertaken, as laid out in the EU Clinical Trials Directive [8].

Approval of research involving children by the institutional review board (IRB) requires particular attention to the assessment of risks and benefits, and this assessment has implications for the level of authorization.

Briefly, researchers must identify (and the IRB must confirm) the category of the proposed research. There are four potential categories (outlined in **Table 2**). As can be seen from this table, the assessment of risk relies on the concept of 'minimal risk'. Minimal risk is defined as being those risks for which "the probability and magnitude of harm or discomfort… are not greater in and of themselves than those normally encountered in daily life or during the performance of routine physical or psychological examinations or tests" (45 CFR 46.102) [2]. For example, studies that involve noninvasive psychological testing to investigate cognitive patterns in psychiatric disorders might fit into this category.

Some have expressed concern over whether this definition is specific enough to give guidance, as it might allow sick children to be exposed to more risks than healthy children, and there are risks that we do not want children to face even

Section of 45 CFR 46 referred to	Risks and benefits	Requirements	Examples*
46.406	No greater than minimal risk	Assent of child and permission of one parent	Survey questionnaires Single blood draws Non-invasive testing (eg, X-ray, skin or scalp culture)
46.405	More than minimal risk, but prospect of direct benefit to child	Anticipated benefit is at least as favorable as that of available alternatives Assent of child and permission of one parent	Phase II or III trials Invasive testing Repeated blood sampling Some psychological testing
46.406	More than minimal risk and no prospect of direct benefit, but likely to yield generalizable knowledge about the subject's disorder	Minor increase over minimal risk Research procedures are similar to those the subject would normally experience in expected medical, social, or educational situations Assent of child and permission of both parents	Repeated blood samples for pharmacokinetic studies Some Phase I trials Repeat of familiar invasive procedure, such as bronchoscopy
46.407	Research not covered in 46.404, .405, or .406 (ie, more than a minor increase in risk and no prospect of direct benefit)	Research must present a reasonable opportunity to further the understanding, prevention, or alleviation of a serious problem affecting the health or welfare of children Assent of child and permission of both parents Review and approval by a panel of experts assembled by the Secretary of HHS and public review	Some Phase I trials Biopsy not needed for treatment

Table 2. Categories of pediatric research (45 CFR 46, subpart D). CFR: Code of Federal Regulations; HHS: US Department of Health and Human Services.
*The actual categorization depends on precise details regarding risks and benefits.

though they might encounter these in everyday life [9]. Therefore, for each protocol, researchers and IRB members must determine the exact level of risk and benefit that is presented by participation.

The rules are intended to provide increasing levels of protection as the ratio of risk to benefit increases. For example, research that is categorized as 46.404 and 46.405 requires the permission of only one parent, while that classed as 46.406 or 46.407 requires the permission of both parents. Research that is categorized as 46.407 – ie, that which would present substantial risk with no prospect of direct benefit – would rarely be justified and would require federal review by a panel assembled by the Secretary of HHS, as well as being subjected to public review.

In addition to establishing the risk/benefit category, research protocols involving children must address how risk will be minimized and justify the inclusion of this vulnerable population. For example, protocols that require multiple blood samples to be taken over a short period of time, such as pharmacokinetic studies, should specify that indwelling catheters will be used to avoid the need for repeated venipuncture. In general, it is expected that, if possible, new drugs or procedures should first be tested on animals and then on adults before testing in children.

Authorization

Consent, Assent, and Permission

All of the issues of risk and their justification must be considered in the early stages of study design in order to justify any involvement of children in research. Assuming that these issues can be addressed and the research can be established as justifiable, the issue of informed consent is the next source of complexity.

The basis for the expectations in this area are, again, the same as with any human subject. Fundamental respect for the person requires researchers to forego involving persons without freely given informed consent. Given the restrictions on the intellectual capacity of children, proxy consent (more appropriately referred to as 'permission') is accepted.

As with adult subjects, the IRB can waive the requirement for informed consent and classify the project as 'exempt' if it involves only educational testing, the analysis of existing data, public benefit service programs, or food taste and quality evaluations [2].

The requirement for parental permission is relatively straightforward in that it mirrors the requirement for informed consent from competent adults. That is, the informed consent process and documentation must include all of the components that are required for consenting competent adults, eg, an explanation of procedures, risks and benefits, and costs.

Assent
In addition to obtaining informed consent from parents, researchers must usually also obtain the affirmative (ie, explicit) agreement of the child who will be the actual research subject; this is referred to as 'assent'. This means that the child must receive an explanation of the research and agree to participate; the mere absence of an objection is not sufficient to constitute assent.

There are three situations in which the requirement to obtain the agreement of the child can be waived:

- if the child is not capable of giving meaningful assent
  (eg, the child's age or physical condition renders him/her
  incapable of any comprehension of even simplified explanations)
- if the research offers the prospect of direct and significant
  benefits that would not be available outside of the research
  (eg, an experimental treatment for a serious or life-threatening
  condition for which there are no known effective
  nonexperimental therapies)
- if the research is considered exempt from the requirement for
  informed consent (as described previously, eg, the analysis
  of existing data)

Neither the HHS federal regulations nor the FDA regulations specify the exact age at which a child is deemed to be capable of giving assent. Investigators must take into account the physical age, maturity, and psychological state of the individual subject.

The IRB is expected to evaluate whether the proposed plan for obtaining or waiving assent is justified, including the specific way in which written or verbal assent is to be documented. Therefore, protocols involving children must address the assent plan and include a copy of any information sheets provided to children or parents, as well as assent documents.

Assent is a complex idea, both morally and practically. The moral justification for requiring that children agree to participate before involving them in research stems from the respect that is due to them as human beings, without regard to their maturity or cognitive status. The waiver of this requirement, in situations in which the child's health or wellbeing can be significantly and positively affected by participation, stems from our duty as a society and as parents to act in the best interests of the child.

In situations in which the parents and treating clinicians perceive an overriding obligation to provide experimental treatment, it is not appropriate to attempt to solicit agreement from the child [10], although it is always appropriate to provide the child with explanations. These sometimes competing considerations – of the duty to respect the child's wishes and the duty to provide needed treatment – mean that each specific situation must be evaluated individually in order to know what is required.

In practical terms, assent is complex because it is not clear how best to determine when children are capable of understanding and giving meaningful agreement. In addition, the best format for providing explanations, the exact amount of information that should be provided, and methods to assess understanding are not known. Each of these topics must be considered in the design and implementation of consent/assent procedures.

Judging Capacity

Federal regulations do not define the age at which the assent of the child subject is required. This is reasonable given the wide variation in cognitive capacity and maturity of children. A general norm that has been developed suggests that children below the age of 6 or 7 years are not capable of understanding research or providing meaningful authorization for research. Children between 6 and 13/14 years of age are generally thought to be capable of reading assent forms that explain research in simplified terms, including the research's purpose, procedures, and risks [11,12]. Children of 14 years of age and above may be able to read and sign the same consent forms that are signed by their parents.

As with adults, many other factors must also be considered for each individual subject and each protocol. Parental views regarding the child's reading level, observations of other healthcare providers or teachers regarding the maturity of the child, and considerations related to cultural norms regarding the child's decision-making independence can all provide relevant information that should be taken into account in deciding both the appropriateness of seeking assent and the form of assent (written or oral).

Voluntary Nature of Participation

The traditional concept of 'informed consent' has two components:

- the informational requirement
- the volitional or consensual requirement

Because of practical difficulties with crafting a meaningful document or script to explain research to children, there has been a tendency to focus on this issue. However, the challenge of assuring that the assent of the child is freely given also warrants close attention.

Children are influenced by the authority figures in their lives. This certainly includes parents and might also include physicians, teachers, and other healthcare professionals, such as nurses or counselors. Because of this, researchers should be alert to the possibility that children might be reluctant to express dissent when these authority figures are present. This suggests that there might be situations in which it is appropriate to talk with the child alone and provide an opportunity for the child to ask questions or express doubts without his/her parents being present. On the other hand, young children rely on the guidance and assurance of their parents and it may be reasonable for parents to be reluctant to allow researchers with whom they are not familiar to talk to their children without their presence.

While there is no accepted guideline regarding when parents should be present or absent during assent discussions, researchers should be alert to any subtle indication that the potential subject is uncomfortable with the idea of participation. This is particularly important if the research involves sensitive topics such as mental health issues, sexuality, or drug use.

The principles and guidelines for obtaining freely given consent from adults are useful in planning the approach to obtaining assent from children. Most importantly, the responsibility to obtain assent should be thought of as a process, not an event. Children, just as adults, require time to think about the information given to them, to ask questions, and to change their mind.

Compensation

The issue of compensation presents an additional threat to the voluntary nature of participation. Compensation is a controversial subject in all research. The permissibility, and possibly even obligation, to provide some form of compensation for the time and trouble associated with research procedures is generally offered as the strongest justification for providing monetary payments or gifts to research subjects.

The well-recognized danger is that large payments can act as inducements, particularly to vulnerable groups such as the poor, and thus they constitute a powerful influence on decision-making that reduces the voluntary nature of participation. Children are thought to be particularly vulnerable to the promise of receiving money or desired gifts, and there is a worry that parents may be unduly influenced to allow their children to bear the burdens of research by the promise of monetary compensation.

Recommendations for how to deal with this issue in pediatric research have included [6,13]:

- prohibition of any compensation
- only telling children about compensation after assent has been obtained
- insisting that all payments should go to the child rather than his/her parents
- making payment in the form of child-appropriate gifts

While there is no consensus and no federal rules about this issue, some generally accepted guidelines are outlined in **Table 3**.

Assent Forms

Preparing an age-appropriate and meaningful assent form to be read and signed by a child, or drafting a script to be used in talking with a child, is challenging. It requires not only familiarity with the research protocol, but also an authentic commitment to the respectful involvement of the child and an understanding of the child's developmental stage. Some of the major questions to be considered when drafting the document or script are outlined in **Table 4**.

• Compensation should be provided to the parties that bear the burdens of participation; this generally means that the child-subject should receive the compensation. If, however, parents have to take time off work or pay transportation costs then it is reasonable to include them in the compensation scheme. • Monetary compensation for the time of parents and older children should be proportional to minimum wage payments, as is the case for adult subjects.	• Compensation for young children should be in the form of age-appropriate gifts (eg, coupons for video stores, movie tickets, child/infant supplies such as diapers, or gift certificates for children's stores) and should be limited to the value appropriate for a 'thank you' gift. • Protocols for IRB review should provide justification for the choice of compensation.

Table 3. Some generally accepted guidelines for dealing with compensation in pediatric research. IRB: institutional review board.

• What are children of this age likely to want to know? • What will children of this age be able to understand?	• What is this age group's decision-making capacity? • What information is important for a potential subject to have in order to make a decision?

Table 4. Some of the major questions to be considered when drafting an assent form or script for children [14].

Although there have been recommendations for the standardization of the topics and terminology in assent forms and national guidelines on this issue [6], this has not yet occurred. Therefore, investigators must rely on familiar general principles when constructing assent scripts or forms. These include the following:

- Use terminology with which the child is likely to be familiar, rather than standard adult verbiage (see **Table 5** for examples).
- Most assent forms should include the following components: the reason why the study is being done; what the child will experience (eg, blood samples, questionnaires); any anticipated benefits of the study; assurances about the voluntary nature of participation; and, if appropriate, how confidentiality will be ensured.
- Keep the assent form to one or two pages at most. Do not include all the elements required in an adult informed consent document (eg, background information, privacy authorization, discussions about liability).

> **Keep terminology simple**
>
> "The doctor will stick you with a needle and this will hurt for just a minute," rather than "We will draw a blood sample; this may cause minimal brief pain."
>
> "The nurse will ask you to pee in a bottle," rather than "We will collect a sample of your urine."
>
> **Use general summaries**
>
> "We want to find out more about what happens when kids like you have trouble breathing," rather than "The purpose of this study is to measure the levels of certain chemicals in the blood of children with asthma in order to..."
>
> **Reassure the child that they do not have to participate**
>
> "If you don't want to do this, you don't have to. No one will be mad at you."

Table 5. Tips for ensuring that language is child-friendly.

- Use general summaries of two or three sentences, rather than details that will not be meaningful to a child.
- The assent process (verbal and written) should always include assurance that the child does not have to participate.
- The child should also be assured that he/she can ask questions now or later, and can change his/her mind at any time.

In addition, several other aspects of the assent process must be addressed. These include the choice of presenter, the timing and location, and whether the child's parents will be present. It is preferable to have someone who is skilled and comfortable in talking with children present the assent form or talk to the child; this may not be a primary investigator.

The conversation should take place in a quiet area, and at a time when the child is not distracted, tired, or uncomfortable from having undergone other procedures. Comprehension should be assessed by asking the child to tell the presenter what he/she understands about what will happen. The child should be offered the opportunity to talk about the research again at a later time. These guidelines are similar to the considerations that are relevant when seeking consent or permission from adults, and reinforce the importance of viewing assent as a process rather than an event.

Remaining Issues and Questions

A number of issues regarding IRB authorization to enroll children in research are controversial and remain unresolved. These include:

- more precise definitions of 'minimal' and 'minor increase over minimal risk' [6,15]
- the need for child advocates in research involving more than minimal risk [6]
- clarification of methods to assess capacity to give assent [16]
- procedures for authorizing the participation of children who are wards of the state or court

Research involving adolescents is particularly problematic [11,17]. State and national laws vary both in how they define special classes of adolescents who have legal authority to consent to medical treatment (eg, emancipated minors and mature minors) and the type of medical treatment that can be accessed without parental permission (eg, treatment for sexually transmitted diseases, contraception, treatment of substance abuse). Most state and national laws do not address whether adolescents can consent to research on these topics.

Further adding to the complexity, FDA rules differ from 45 CFR 46 with regard to the waiver of parental permission for research. Federal regulations (45 CFR 46.408[c]) allow for a waiver in circumstances in which parental permission would be inappropriate, such as investigations relating to child abuse [2]. However, in adopting most of the provisions of 45 CFR 46, the FDA specifically omitted this section and so requires investigators to obtain parental permission in all cases. Therefore, investigators who propose to enroll adolescents in studies in which parental permission might be problematic are advised to consider their specific state laws and to obtain guidance from their IRB as well as regulatory agencies before designing authorization (assent or permission) procedures.

Conclusion

This chapter has presented considerations that must be addressed when enrolling children in research. As a vulnerable population, children are protected from research risks both by restrictions on the degree of risk to which they can be exposed and by the requirement that parental permission must be obtained before enrolling minors. The moral obligation of respect for persons imposes the further requirement that the explicit assent of children to participate be obtained before involving them in research procedures.

While the ethical basis for requiring assent is clear, designing effective and meaningful approaches to acquire this is a complex challenge that warrants careful and thoughtful attention.

References

1. National Commission for the Protection of Human Subjects of Biomedical and Behavioral Research. Belmont Report: Ethical Principles and Guidelines for the Protection of Human Subjects of Research. Washington, DC: US Government Printing Office, 1979.

2. Department of Health and Human Services (45 CFR 46 subpart D). Additional protections for children involved as subjects in research. Fed Regist 1983;48:9,814-20. Revised in: Fed Regist 1991;56:28,032.

3. US Department of Health and Human Services, Food and Drug Administration. Additional safeguards for children in clinical investigations of FDA-regulated products. Interim rule. Fed Regist 2001;66:20,589-600.

4. International Conference on Harmonisation of Technical Requirements for Registration of Pharmaceuticals for Human Use. Available from: www.ich.org. Accessed November 21, 2004.

5. UK Medical Research Council. Available from: www.mrc.ac.uk. Accessed November 21, 2004.

6. Statement before the Institute of Medicine Committee on Clinical Research Involving Children. Participation and Protection of Children in Clinical Research Presented by Christine Gleason (on behalf of the Society for Pediatric Research and the American Pediatric Society) to the National Academy of Sciences on July 9, 2003. Available from: www.aps-spr.org/Public_Policy/2003_Docs/IOM0709.htm. Accessed November 12, 2004.

7. The Nuremberg Code. In: Trials of War Criminals before the Nuremberg Military Tribunals under Control Council Law No. 10. Washington, DC: US Government Printing Office, 1949;2:181-2. Available from: ohsr.od.nih.gov/guidelines/nuremberg.html. Accessed November 17, 2004.

8. EU Clinical Trials Directive. Available from: www.europa.eu.int/eur-lex/en/search_lif.html. Accessed February 15, 2005.

9. Ross LF, Do Healthy children deserve greater protection in medical research? J Pediatr 2003;142:108-2.

10. Committee on Bioethics, American Academy of Pediatrics. Informed consent, parental permission, and assent in pediatric practice. Pediatrics 1995;95:314-7.

11. Santelli JS, Smith Rogers A, Rosenfeld WD, et al. Guidelines for adolescent health research: A position paper of the society for adolescent medicine. J Adolesc Health 2003;33:396-409.

12. Simar MR, Johnson VA. Pediatric informed consent. Applied Clinical Trials 2002 (July):46-55.

13. Wendler D, Rackoff JE, Emanuel EJ, et al. The ethics of paying for children's participation in research. J Pediatr 2002;141:166-171.

14. Kenny N, Miller P. Comment: Research involving children: Clarifying roles and authority. J Clin Ethics 2000;11:151-6.

15. Robinson WM. Ethical issues in pediatric research. J Clin Ethics 2000;11:145-50.

16. Olechnowicz JQ, Eder M, Simon C, et al. Assent observed: children's involvement in leukemia treatment and research discussions. Pediatrics 2002;109:806-14.

17. Office for Protection from Research Risks, National Institutes of Health, US Department of Health and Human Services. Protecting Human Research Subjects. Institutional Review Board Guidebook. Washington, DC: US Government Printing Office, 1993.

Chapter 7

Study Implementation and Start-up

Belinda Lees
Jean Booth

Introduction

As a clinical research coordinator (CRC), you may be involved in a number of different types of research study and your role will vary depending on the study. However, many of the procedures and principles that you need to follow will be common to all. This chapter is primarily concerned with the processes involved in the successful start-up and implementation of a research study.

Types of Study

Research studies can be performed in just one institution (single center) or in many different institutions (multicenter), which may be all in one country or multinational. Studies can take place in different settings – eg, primary care units, hospitals, nursing homes, or in the community. Studies can also be of various designs, the most common being observational studies or randomized studies (see **Table 1**).

Pharmaceutical studies can be described using the US Food and Drug Administration (FDA) classification for the development of a drug in humans (see **Table 2**).

Study design	Description	Type of study
Case report	Interesting or relevant aspects of a single case (eg, an atypical reaction after a new medication).	Observational
Case series	A group of case reports comprising similar observations, or where similar treatments or procedures have been used (usually in consecutive patients).	Observational
Cross-sectional survey	The selection of a particular population or cohort. Within this cohort, patient characteristics, treatments, and the prevalence of disease are then documented.	Observational
Case control	These studies identify individuals with a particular disease or outcome (the case) and those without it (the control). Comparisons of possible etiological factors in subjects' histories are then carried out.	Observational
Cohort studies	Groups of people are defined who do not have the disease or outcome of interest, but who have, or do not have, particular risk factors. These subjects are then followed to compare the incidence of a disease or outcome of interest between different groups.	Observational
Clinical trials	These are studies that evaluate a therapeutic, invasive, surgical, or care management intervention by using a process of randomization, ie, each subject is allocated to a treatment by chance. This allows treatment groups to be balanced for known and unknown variables that may influence the disease process and response to treatment.	Randomized

Table 1. Examples of study designs.

Study Organization

In multicenter studies, there is usually a coordinating center with whom the individual sites are required to liaise at each stage of the study. The coordinating center can be an academic group, contract research organization, or an industry sponsor. Each center will also have a local investigator, often called the principal investigator, who takes responsibility for the study at that site.

Phase	Description
I	Used for the first investigation of a new drug in humans (often called 'first into man' studies)
	The pharmacokinetic and pharmacologic effects of a drug may be investigated, including its dose–response and side-effects
	Conducted in small numbers of subjects who are usually healthy volunteers
II	Designed using information gained from Phase I studies
	Closely controlled and monitored studies conducted in small numbers of patients (<100)
	Provide preliminary efficacy and safety data
III	Conducted to demonstrate the safety and efficacy of a drug
	Involve hundreds or thousands of patients
	Phase IIIb studies are carried out to investigate new indications for already licensed drugs
IV	Surveillance in many thousands of patients to identify less common adverse effects
	Post-marketing studies to investigate the use of a drug in special populations of patients

Table 2. Phases of drug development.

Studies usually have a trial steering committee (TSC), which is responsible for the scientific content and conduct of the study. The TSC is usually comprised of:

- a chairperson, who may also be the principal investigator
- other investigators, who are specialists within the clinical area of investigation
- a statistician or expert in clinical trials methodology
- an operational expert in clinical trials

The size of the TSC is usually proportional to the size of the study.

The TSC appoints a data monitoring committee (DMC), which oversees the safety of the study. The DMC is generally composed of three or four members who are independent of the trial, and includes a statistician and clinical experts within the area of investigation. Studies may also have a clinical events review committee (CERC), comprised of clinical experts in the disease of interest, which adjudicates

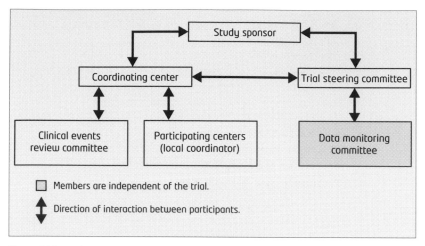

Figure 1. The typical organization of a multicenter clinical trial.

on clinical events to ensure that they meet the definitions given in the protocol. The CERC is blinded to the treatment allocation and members are not allowed to adjudicate events for their own patients. A typical organizational structure for a multicenter clinical trial is shown in **Figure 1**.

Taking Part in a Study

Study Site Selection
Study start-up usually includes a site visit, where the coordinating center performs a feasibility assessment to determine a participating center's facilities, access to patients, patient management, and the number of patients with the disease under investigation. At this point, you may be required to review the study protocol and sign a confidentiality agreement.

Participating centers and local investigators are likely to be selected on the basis of their experience in conducting research, as well as their experience of the disease or condition under investigation. The coordinating center will want to be satisfied that participating centers will be able to enroll sufficient patients for the study within a defined time period. Therefore, you may be asked to complete a screening log to determine the numbers of eligible patients at your center. A pilot study will sometimes be performed to establish the feasibility of a study. The coordinating

Scientific	Does the study address a question of clinical and scientific relevance?
	Is the study likely to achieve its scientific goals?
	Are there any ethical considerations (eg, any risk to subjects)?
	What impact will the study have on patients (eg, will extra investigations be required)?
Practical	Can the sample size be achieved in the available time?
	Are the eligibility criteria realistic?
	What are the procedures for data collection and processing?
	Do you have the necessary staff to perform the trial?
	Are there any special investigations/equipment required?
Financial	What are the local costs of participating (eg, pharmacy and laboratory costs, cost of staff training)?
	What will be the cost of staff for time spent conducting the study at your center?
	What is the payment schedule?

Table 3. Summary of scientific, practical, and financial considerations of a study.

center will also want to establish that the investigator has skilled and dedicated staff, including a CRC, to run the study at the center.

Protocol Assessment

The first task for the CRC is to assess the scientific, practical, and financial implications of the study. These are summarized in Table 3.

You should read the protocol and other study documents carefully, and discuss these in detail with the local investigator and your colleagues at the institution. You should consult with appropriate colleagues, eg, the pharmacy regarding the study drug, theatre managers regarding devices, and laboratory staff regarding blood or pathology specimens.

It is essential that you understand the clinical and scientific importance of the study, not least so that you are able to explain the study clearly to others. It is particularly important for you to determine if the study is likely to be acceptable to patients and what impact the study might have on them in terms of time, commitment, risk, and inconvenience.

You should carefully consider the practical aspects of the study, such as:

- How will concurrent studies and your (and your colleagues') clinical workload affect your ability to recruit patients within the specified time?
- Are the eligibility criteria realistic for your patient population?
- How will you screen and recruit patients?
- Will the timing of follow-up visits fit in with clinic times or required tests?
- Do you have adequate office space where you can discuss the study confidentially with patients and consent/examine patients?
- What special procedures are required for the study (eg, collecting, storing, and sending samples to a central laboratory)?
- Are there particular tests that require specific equipment to be ordered?
- How are data going to be collected (eg, on case report forms [CRFs], or by electronic data collection) and sent to the coordinating center (eg, by fax)?
- Do you have sufficient office space to complete paperwork, enter data, and store study documents?
- Do you have appropriate facilities (eg, fax, telephone, and computers)?
- How is the randomization/unblinding service to be operated?
- What are the procedures for reporting serious adverse events (SAEs)?
- Will staff need to be recruited and/or trained for the study?

Finally, you should consider the financial aspects of the study:

- Is the payment schedule per patient?
- Is the payment schedule dependent on 'clean' data (ie, data that are free from edit queries)?
- Does the payment schedule include patient expenses?
- Is there funding for special equipment or tests?
- Are the pharmacy costs adequate?
- Will there be shipping costs for samples, tapes, and CDs?
- What are the payment arrangements if a patient discontinues?

Item	Amount
Institutional overheads	
Recruitment, salary, and training costs for staff working on the study	
Regulatory submission costs	
Ethical submission costs	
Institutional review of protocol and agreements	
Pharmacy review of protocol, storage, and dispensing of study drug	
Study materials, eg, case report forms, protocols, study summaries	
Patient materials, eg, patient diaries, drug dispensers	
Advertising for patients	
Patient travel expenses	
Study-specific blood tests, measurements, and scans	
Shipping costs for samples/scans	
Study-specific equipment (the sponsor may provide or loan this)	
Office equipment, eg, filing cabinets	
Stationery and postage	
Telephone, fax, computer, and printer	
Travel costs to meetings	
Contingency sum (allow 10% for unexpected expenses)	
Total	

Table 4. Summary of items to consider when planning the study budget.

A summary of some of the considerations when budgeting for a study is shown in **Table 4**.

Investigator and Coordinator Meetings

Most multicenter studies will involve regular meetings between the investigator and the CRCs. These meetings usually take place:

- at the start of the study – to discuss the protocol and practical aspects of the trial

• The final, original, signed protocol and any protocol amendments	• The patient consent form
	• Any literature used for recruitment (eg, advertisements)
• Any documents requiring patient involvement (eg, patient diaries, questionnaires)	• The investigator payment schedule
	• Information on patient payment or compensation
• The investigator's brochure and any safety information	• Regulatory documents pertaining to the investigational product (where applicable)
• The investigator's CV/résumé	
• The patient information sheet, tailored to local requirements	

Table 5. Documents usually required to be submitted to the institutional review board/independent ethics committee.

- during the study – to discuss progress and any problems
- at the end of the study – to present and discuss the results

These meetings are a good opportunity to meet the other CRCs involved in the study and to share and resolve any problems. For some studies, an investigator meeting, prior to study start-up, will take the place of a site initiation visit. Site initiation can also take the form of training by telephone.

Ethical and Regulatory Approval

All studies must be submitted to an institutional review board (IRB) or independent ethics committee (IEC) for approval before taking place at an institution. You should determine how frequently your IRB/IEC meets and their exact requirements. The usual documents to be submitted to the IRB/IEC are summarized in **Table 5**.

If you are performing a study where an investigational product is being given or a device used, appropriate regulatory approval from the Medicines and Healthcare Products Regulatory Agency, FDA, European Medicines Agency, or national regulatory body must be obtained before starting the study.

Indemnity and Financial Agreements

Before the study starts at your center, you need to ensure that insurance/indemnity agreements and a signed agreement between your institution and the sponsor are in place. Insurance/indemnity agreements provide insurance to indemnify (ie, to secure against liability) the investigator and to compensate the patient in the event of a trial-related injury. The details of the indemnity agreement will vary from study to study. The signed agreement between your institution and the sponsor should include details of the parties' responsibilities and the financial agreement.

The research services department and/or financial managers at your institution will need to review the protocol and financial agreement and give authorization to proceed. This process is often performed in parallel with the IRB/IEC application.

Study Organization

Establish the logistics of the study at your institution. You may find the following checklist helpful:

- Liaise with colleagues as early as possible to discuss the study protocol and procedures on a one-to-one basis or in group training sessions, whichever is most appropriate.
- Establish who will screen, consent, and randomize patients. Ensure that an authorized person is always available for these procedures.
- Determine if only the investigator can consent patients or if other personnel delegated by the investigator may do this. This is particularly important in studies involving acute admissions.
- Identify where in your institution the patient will be seen.
- For follow-up visits, establish who will see patients and perform study-related tests, procedures, or measurements. You may find that a flow chart is helpful to show the tests that are required at each visit and any timelines for visit dates.
- Identify who will take responsibility for any samples, scans, or tests that are to be sent to a central laboratory (where applicable).
- Determine who will complete CRFs and study documentation, and who will report SAEs.
- Ensure that staff are in place and appropriately trained.
- Order special equipment and/or test kits, and liaise with the pharmacy about the drugs and/or devices that will be used in the study.
- Arrange space: in which patient interviews and measurements can be carried out; for the completion of documents; in which computers, fax machines, and telephones can be set up; and for the safe storage of documents.

• The final, original, signed protocol and any amendments	• A specimen copy of the patient consent form
• The letter of approval from the institutional review board/ independent ethics committee and any correspondence	• A specimen copy of the patient information sheet and any information to be given to the subject
• A copy of the regulatory approval (the sponsor will provide this, if applicable)	• The patient recruitment advertisement (if applicable)
• The letter of indemnity (for insurance purposes)	• A specimen copy of the case report form
• Signed agreements between all parties (including financial agreements)	• The list of laboratory normal ranges, methods, and accreditation/ calibration certificates
• CVs/résumés for the investigator, study team, laboratory director, and pharmacist (if applicable)	• The trial training/initiation visit report
	• Instructions for use of the study drug or device (if not in protocol)
• The list of authorized signatories	• The method for emergency unblinding
• The investigator's brochure	• Shipping records for the investigational product and its certificate of analysis (where applicable)

Table 6. Essential study documents.

- Prepare advertising materials (eg, on posters, television, radio, and the Internet, and patient support pamphlets). Ensure that such materials have received IRB/IEC approval before use.
- Design and print notepaper, logos, and newsletters, and set up a Web page.

Training

Prior to the commencement of the study, the coordinating center will usually perform a training visit to your center. You should ensure that all personnel who will be involved in the study can attend (eg, pharmacy and laboratory staff) and that the essential study documents are available for review (**Table 6**).

The coordinating center will want to ensure that the personnel at your center are trained in the study's procedures and measurements, and in Good Clinical Practice. The coordinating center might also wish to visit your center's laboratories or pharmacy to check the facilities and documentation.

Following the training visit, you should ensure that you are fully conversant with all study procedures, including:

Use the start-up phase to increase awareness of the study by the following methods:
- put up posters in your institution summarizing the study
- ensure colleagues are familiar with the eligibility criteria
- hold lunchtime seminars to disseminate information about the study to clinical colleagues
- talk to patient support groups
- submit articles to patient support magazines (ensure that you have institutional review board/independent ethics committee approval before doing this)

Table 7. Increasing study awareness.

- eligibility criteria
- recruitment procedures
- the randomization method
- how the study drug is to be dispensed, or the study device used
- how to perform unblinding (if applicable)
- how the CRF and adverse event forms are to be completed
- the method for reporting SAEs
- study measurements
- how samples are to be transported
- Good Clinical Practice

Increasing Study Awareness

Use the start-up phase to increase awareness of the study. Some tips to assist you are summarized in **Table 7**.

Planning Your Time

To perform a study effectively, it is essential that you are able to dedicate yourself to the study. The amount of time that you will need to spend will depend on the complexity of the study and the number of patients to be enrolled. Your input will almost certainly vary throughout the life-cycle of the study, and the following guidelines may be helpful.

Start-up Phase

This will be a very busy time for you – allow 3–6 months for this phase. You will perform the following tasks:

- reviewing the protocol
- IRB/IEC submission
- regulatory submission

- recruiting and training staff
- purchasing of equipment
- organizing the study drug or device (if applicable)

Recruitment of Patients

Allow for the recruitment period specified in the protocol. This phase will also be very busy for you, as you will need to ensure that you are available for all appropriate clinics or patient appointments so that you can screen all potentially eligible patients. Screening logs will assist you in estimating the time that recruitment is likely to take at your center.

Follow-up of Patients

Allow for the follow-up measurement period specified in the protocol. You may be very busy during this phase if there are complex or frequent follow-up measurements, but less so if follow-up is to be performed by telephone, or by tracking notes or events. You will also be required to report adverse events.

Close-out Phase

This phase will take up to 3 months and will often be very time consuming, as you will need to resolve edit queries and clean data.

Reporting of Study

This phase will take up to 3 months and will usually be less busy. However, you may be involved in the analysis of the data, presenting the findings, and writing the final report and manuscript.

Conclusion

As the CRC, you are key to the successful implementation and start-up of the study. Your role might vary, but you should try to be involved right from the beginning of the start-up phase when the site selection process is occurring:

- assess the protocol for scientific, practical, and financial implications
- attend investigator meetings
- submit ethical and regulatory approvals

- coordinate indemnity and financial agreements
- become fully conversant in the study procedures
- increase study awareness
- organize the study at your center and your workload

Careful planning in the study start-up phase will help to ensure the successful conduct of a study.

Useful Web Sites

For US Sites/Studies:

www.fda.gov
US Food and Drug Administration (FDA)

www.fda.gov/cdrh
Center for Devices and Radiological Health

www.fda.gov/medwatch
MedWatch: FDA Safety and Adverse Event Reporting

For UK Sites/Studies:

www.corec.org.uk
Central Office for Research Ethics Committees

www.mhra.gov.uk
Medicines and Healthcare Products Regulatory Agency

www.mrc.ac.uk
Medical Research Council

http://www.dh.gov.uk/PolicyAndGuidance/ResearchAndDevelopment/fs/en
Department of Health: research and development pages

www.invo.org.uk
INVOLVE: promoting public involvement in NHS, public health, and social care research

www.ct-toolkit.ac.uk
Clinical Trials Toolkit (practical help for researchers performing clinical trials, from the Department of Health and Medical Research Council)

Other International Sites:

www.emea.eu.int
European Medicines Agency

www.nihs.go.jp/pmdec/outline.htm
Japan's Pharmaceutical and Medical Device Evaluation Centre

Chapter 8

Recruitment and Retention of Research Subjects

Rebecca Mister

Nicola Delahunty

Aviva Grosbard

Introduction

Subject recruitment and retention are major factors in running and completing a successful clinical trial. Timelines can be tight due to both financial issues and the responsibility of answering a scientifically important question. Meeting recruitment targets is one of the keys to achieving the projected timelines.

Therefore, when designing a trial, consideration needs to be given to how subjects will be recruited, as well as to the science behind the protocol. Clinical research subjects are not easy to find; a 2001 report from CenterWatch stated that over 85% of all medical research studies that were completed experienced enrollment delays, and 34% were delayed for more than 1 month [1].

When reviewing an offer to participate in a clinical trial, you need to consider whether you see enough eligible subjects in your institution. Inevitably, some target populations will be met more quickly than others – eg, recruitment times have been shown to be two to three times quicker for the therapeutic classes of anti-infective and antiviral treatments compared with those for cardiac therapies [2].

Question	Explanation
What is the severity of the condition being studied?	Will your subjects be found in physicians' surgeries or will they be hospital in-patients or out-patients?
Is the condition acute or chronic?	Subjects with acute diseases are likely to be admitted as hospital in-patients
Is there a specific location where you may find this subject population?	For example, you are most likely to find renal subjects in a dialysis unit and postmyocardial infarction subjects in a rehabilitation clinic

Table 1. Questions to help you to identify where to look for eligible subjects.

To effectively recruit subjects into a research study, it is essential that you, as the clinical research coordinator (CRC), understand and have confidence in the purpose of the study. The protocol will summarize the specific aims of the study – the inclusion/exclusion criteria, any procedures involved, and the risks and benefits to subjects – establishing a foundation for the informed consent process.

Estimation of Subject Numbers

The inclusion/exclusion criteria serve as the starting point for targeting potential subjects. Posters summarizing inclusion/exclusion criteria can act as a prompt for staff at your institution to contact the study team if they see a suitable subject. Remember that any such materials/information will usually need to be approved by your institutional review board (IRB)/independent ethics committee (IEC) prior to use.

Some hospitals have large research teams who review the eligibility of all subjects admitted for participation in a trial. At other sites, there may only be the principal investigator (PI) and CRC managing one or more trials: in this case, you might be responsible for identifying potential study subjects. Three important questions that will enable a focused approach to looking for eligible subjects are given in **Table 1**, while site-specific methods for facilitating screening and recruitment once your site has commenced participation in a study are provided in **Table 2**.

There is an almost invariable phenomenon called the 'funnel effect', whereby a pool of potential subjects who are contacted about entering a clinical trial becomes progressively smaller as it passes through successive screens and the informed consent process [3]. The funnel effect illustrates the progressive shrinking of the patient population prior to enrolling in a trial.

Method	Explanation
Increase the screening area	Review subject notes and hospital databases
	Visit patient areas (eg, wards, clinics) daily, if possible
	Review screening logs from previous trials
Ensure colleagues are aware of the study	Regularly present the study at education meetings at your site
	Regularly distribute information about the study (ie, newsletters, posters) - remember that ethical approval is required for this material
	Consider presenting the study at local research meetings
Use advertising and marketing	Target subject support groups
	Write articles
	Consider giving presentations to support groups

Table 2. Methods of increasing recruitment rates.

The end result of the funnel effect is the number of subjects who enter the clinical trial, and this number can be expressed as a percentage yield of those screened or initially contacted. It has been stated that a general loss of 90% of subjects can be anticipated, although the screening yield probably depends on the type of trial population sought. The yield is primarily related to the inclusion criteria *plus* the protocol *plus* the motivation of subjects to enroll [3].

This funnel effect could be extended to include dropout and discontinuation during the clinical trial, but these events are separate and relate to the clinical trial and not to the process of patient recruitment. Typically, subjects either dropout on their own or are discontinued by the investigator. If some or all dropouts are to be replaced in a trial then additional subjects must be recruited.

Dropout rates vary widely (1–50%) and are influenced by the following factors:

- outcome measure being used
- length of follow-up
- type of study intervention
- the trial population itself

Dropout and discontinuation rates that are greater than anticipated threaten the successful completion of any clinical trial; anticipated dropout and discontinuation rates must be incorporated in sample size projections to determine the number of patients that should be recruited [3].

Recruitment and the Study Contract

Specific recruitment targets are often detailed in the protocol and, by signing the participation agreement, a site agrees to meet these targets. The site should ensure that it can meet these goals before the contract is signed, as this is a legally binding document. You might be asked to complete a site-specific assessment to see if your site is able to contribute to the study. In some cases recruitment will be competitive: sites can enroll as many subjects as possible until the total sample size has been reached. Sometimes the sponsor will offer a bonus, eg, a gift hamper, for recruiting a predetermined number of subjects. This is a controversial approach that could be viewed as a conflict of interest, as it might encourage the enrollment of subjects for whom participation is not in their best interests.

Payment schedules are confirmed in the contract for each site and are arranged by the sponsor. Subject payments for Phase III and IV studies are related to the cost of each study activity (eg, blood tests, X-rays) and the time taken to perform that activity. In most studies, payments will be made on receipt of 'clean' data (ie, once all data have been received and all queries resolved for a specific visit).

Failure to meet recruitment targets can have serious consequences. If recruitment targets are not met then the study site might not meet budgetary forecasts. This can be very important if subject payments support your salary. If your center is unable to meet recruitment targets then this can also jeopardize future opportunities to participate in other trials managed by that sponsor. Crucially, from a scientific point of view, the inability to meet recruitment targets can lead to delays in completion of the study. Ultimately, this can impede the evaluation of new treatments, leading to slower changes in clinical practice.

It is important to maintain regular contact with the sponsor throughout the study as they will be able to give details of recruitment strategies that have previously been successful. The sponsor might also support recruitment through activities such as nationwide advertising campaigns – any such commitment will be outlined in the contract.

- Pharmacists
- Transfusion specialists
- Ward nurses, doctors, and administrators
- Medical records staff
- Accident and emergency department, and admission wards
- Other departments relevant to your study (eg, X-ray, physiotherapy, dietetics)
- Out-patient staff

Table 3. Examples of the multidisciplinary team members at a clinical research site.

Recruitment

Generating Interest in the Study

It is important to remember that clinical research is a team effort. Before starting a study it is useful to make a list of everyone who will be involved in the trial (see Table 3). Good relationships need to be maintained with all members of the multidisciplinary team at all times in order to enable smooth running at the study site. You will often be responsible for ensuring this.

Once a site has received information about a research study, you should arrange to meet with the relevant people (eg, other research staff, pharmacy and laboratory staff) to discuss the feasibility of the study. The study monitor (clinical research associate) will often have a list of staff members that they need to meet at the initiation visit to ensure that all staff are trained in relevant study procedures (this is a requirement of the International Conference on Harmonisation guidelines for Good Clinical Practice [ICH–GCP]).

When a site has agreed to participate, the study should be presented at a regular meeting (either departmental or institutional), enabling it to reach a wide audience. This increases awareness of the study within the institution and will hopefully generate referrals of potential subjects. Providing refreshments and having the meeting at a convenient time (eg, early morning, lunchtime) can help to maximize attendance, and you should promote the meeting throughout the study site. It is also helpful to visit individual departments (eg, laboratories, pharmacy, medical records department) to meet staff and discuss specific aspects of the study that are relevant to each person. This also creates the basis for a good working relationship.

During the course of the study you might receive regular newsletters from the study sponsor. Once these have been read, distribute them for others to read – this maintains awareness of the study and keeps people informed of progress. Any subject newsletters should be sent to your IRB/IEC for approval before being distributed to subjects. Regular updates of study progress can be posted on your intranet or a study-specific Web site. It is important to update any information regularly – old newsletters can lead to the study becoming ignored by passers-by.

Advertising and Marketing

Advertisements can be used to publicize your study and can help to increase recruitment rates. However, there are many country-specific ethical, regulatory, and institutional regulations surrounding how and where studies can be advertised. Every advertisement needs to be approved by the IRB/IEC before use.

Advertising should be carefully planned as part of the recruitment strategy and can be targeted directly to potential subjects, encouraging them to volunteer, or to physicians so that they will refer suitable subjects. It is important to decide on the characteristics of the target audience (eg, age, race, gender) and to prepare the strategy accordingly. For example, a different strategy would be required when targeting elderly people with heart disease than it would if the target population was young, healthy females.

It is useful to remember that your advertisement might need to target the caregiver as well as the subject (eg, studies in the elderly or in children). Here, both subject and decision-maker profiling are crucial in creating an effective campaign [4]. Discussing a study with subject groups can also yield valuable information when selecting the best methods to use.

Advertising can be costly, and it is useful to look at the potential benefits before deciding on a strategy. Sponsors will often have an advertising program in place. Advertisements can be placed in newspapers, on the radio, TV, or Internet, or delivered as handouts, eg, in doctors' surgeries, out-patient clinics, supermarkets, or other public places. Internet advertising is becoming increasingly popular and is fairly easy to do – a link to study details can be added to subject support group Web sites.

Any advertising campaign should be designed to capture the target audience's imagination and make them want to make contact. An advertisement should be

US Food and Drug Administration (FDA)	
Advertisements should not	• Be unduly coercive
	• State or imply a certainty of benefit, beyond what is outlined in the informed consent document and the study protocol
	• Claim that the treatment under investigation is safe or effective
	• Claim that the treatment under investigation is known to be equivalent or superior to any other treatment
	• Use terms such as 'new treatment,' 'new medication,' or 'new drug' without explaining that the test article is investigational
	• Promise 'free medical treatment' when the intent is only to say that subjects will not be charged for taking part in the investigation
Advertisements may:	• State that subjects will be paid, but should not emphasize the payment or the amount to be paid by means such as bold type.
UK Association of the British Pharmaceutical Industry (ABPI)	
Advertisements should not:	• Imply or express claims of safety or efficacy
	• Place undue emphasis on reimbursement, although mention of reimbursement is permitted
	• Express or imply that the research is FDA or MCA approved
	• Use the term 'new' unless qualified, ie, 'new research medicine,' 'new investigational medicine'
	• Use the compound's name
In addition:	• Care should be taken to ensure that advertisements are in no way promotional for the medicine concerned

Table 4. Advertising guidelines in clinical trial recruitment [6,7]. MCA: Medicines Control Agency.

short and snappy to grab the attention of potential subjects, perhaps with tear-off cards or reply-paid envelopes so that those interested can seek further information [5]. It is important not to offer a 'wonder cure' or to be coercive. Guidelines for advertising are outlined in **Table 4** [6,7].

It is also essential to consider the size of an advertising campaign with regard to the facilities available for handling the responses generated and for scheduling appointments within a timely manner. In 2003, an analysis of prequalified study volunteers for Phase II and III projects found that 13% of potential volunteers did

- Review subject notes
- Visit clinics - general and specialist
- Visit wards and departments, with appropriate approval (ie, from head nurse or department director)
- Review the hospital's databases
- Visit patient areas daily, if possible
- Use advertising
- Target subject support groups by writing articles and/or giving talks
- Respond promptly to any enquiries from potential subjects

Table 5. Some tips for successful subject recruitment.

not enroll because there was no conveniently located investigative site, 14% lost interest following their initial interactions with call center or study staff, and 23% were never randomized because no one contacted them after the initial phone screen [8]. Some tips for successful subject recruitment are given in **Table 5**.

Screening

Potential subjects need to be screened to see if they meet preliminary inclusion criteria before being approached. Once prospective subjects have been identified, you should review the study with each individual. Adequate time should be allowed for the potential subject to review the informed consent document prior to the screening visit. The screening procedure is summarized in **Table 6**.

Some studies require a screening log to be completed, detailing all potential subjects and any reasons for nonenrollment. This enables the coordinating center and research team to monitor study progress. If subject recruitment is proving difficult, the reasons will be documented in the log. If a subject is ineligible for the current study but willing to take part in future research, their information can be included in a 'registry,' providing appropriate consent is obtained. The use of any subject data is covered by certain regulations (eg, the Health Insurance Portability and Accountability Act [HIPAA] in the USA, and the Data Protection Act in the UK) and both sponsors and study site staff must comply with these (see **Chapter 2** for further information about privacy regulations).

- Review subjects' medical notes before approaching them to ensure that they preliminarily meet the eligibility criteria
- Review the results of any tests that could exclude the subject
- Check whether the subject has participated in any other trials (a washout period may be required)
- Carry out any further tests that are required (eg, blood tests, electrocardiograms, X-rays) - this can only be done after the subject has given their written informed consent
- Perform baseline assessments on the subject

Table 6. Summary of the subject screening process.

Protected Health Information

The HIPAA Privacy Rule specifies that a healthcare provider can neither use nor disclose any protected health information (PHI) for research purposes unless the subject has provided, in advance, his/her written authorization for such use or disclosure. This authorization is different from the requirement for informed consent [9]. In the USA, under Title 45, Code of Federal Regulations, Part 164.512(i)(1)(ii), a hospital may permit researchers to view PHI about its subjects for the purposes of preparing a research protocol and recruiting subjects, provided that the researcher demonstrates (either in writing or orally) that [10]:

- the use or disclosure is sought solely to review PHI as necessary to prepare a research protocol, or for similar purposes preparatory to research
- no PHI is to be removed from the hospital by the researcher in the course of the review
- the PHI for which use or access is sought is necessary for the research purposes

The EU Clinical Trials Directive states that subjects should be informed of who will be able to access their clinical trial data, the procedure for handling any identifiable biological samples that have been retained, and plans to anonymize or destroy samples after analysis [11].

Informed Consent

It is important that subjects have adequate time to consider the study, participate in the informed consent process, and do not feel that they have to agree to participate without considering the full implications of taking part in the study because they "don't want to upset the doctor". You are essential to the process as subjects might feel more comfortable asking you questions than asking the physician who is responsible for their care. You are also likely to have more time to spend with the subject to answer any queries they might have. It is essential that the PI is involved in the informed consent process.

There are a number of points to remember when obtaining informed consent for a study:

- Use a quiet place to minimize interruptions.
- Explain the study clearly, including any potential benefits and side effects.
- Inform subjects of any prohibited medications or potential effects on lifestyle (eg, if a drug has sedative effects and driving should be avoided).
- Give the subject the subject information sheet and consent form to read in their own time, and give them ample opportunity to ask questions.
- Explain how participating in the study might differ from routine clinical practice (eg, any additional tests or medications that are required) and ensure that the subject is aware of the duration of follow-up and of all the procedures that will be required.
- Use visual aids such as charts, graphs, and videotapes to improve the subject's understanding of the study.
- Explain that participation is voluntary and that subjects are free to withdraw from the study at any time; emphasize that this will not affect their subsequent medical care, and that this is included on the consent form.
- You might be required to give the subject contact details of an independent adviser who they can talk to about the study, and many institutions now have a contact person with whom subjects can discuss their rights regarding participation is a study.

- IRB/IEC-approved consent forms must be used and must be signed by, and in the presence of, an authorized member of the study team as well as the subject. The subject should be given a signed copy of the information and the consent form. (Note: 45 CFR 46.117 documentation of informed consent states, "A copy shall be given to the person signing the form," whereas ICH–GCP differentiates "signed copy".)

Informed consent is discussed in detail in **Chapter 5**. When signed consent has been obtained and eligibility for enrollment confirmed, you must:

- dispense the study product as specified in the protocol
- show the subject how to use the investigational product (if necessary) and any other study materials (eg, diaries)
- give the subject a study identification card containing details of the study and a contact name and telephone number to use in case of any queries, problems, or emergencies
- write to the subject's family physician informing them of the subject's participation and providing details of the study
- arrange the next follow-up visit (as specified in the protocol) at a convenient time for the subject
- complete the case record form and any other required documentation

Randomization and Blinding

In a randomized controlled trial, randomization of the subject can take place once written informed consent has been obtained and eligibility criteria confirmed. As the CRC, you will carry out the process of randomization as specified in the protocol.

It is usual for everyone involved in the study (including the subject) to be blinded to the treatment allocated, but there will be certain circumstances in which blinding is not possible. In cases of emergency it is always possible to unblind the treatment, but it will usually be sufficient to stop the study medication (in the case of a drug study) and treat the subject as appropriate for the complaint. Maintaining the blind until the end of the study eliminates potential biasing of results.

Compliance and Retention

What Motivates Subjects?

Once a subject has been randomized into a study and has been allocated a treatment it is important to keep them in the study from this point on, both for their safety and for the integrity of the study results. Understanding the reasons that people have for participating should help you to retain subjects. Two of the main motivations are:

- Many subjects will have been ill for a long time and might not be getting much relief from their routine medical care. Such subjects hope that the chance to be involved with a new therapy might improve their condition.
- Many prospective subjects are aware that their own condition might not change, but are willing to take part in the hope that better treatment options will become available in the future, thereby decreasing the suffering of others.

Dispelling the Myths

Often, subjects comment that by taking part in the study they are receiving a better level of care through additional check-ups and, in some instances, tests. While this might be true, it is essential that subjects are aware that their care will not suffer in any way should they decide to withdraw their consent during the study. This point must be included in the subject information sheet and consent form (a requirement of ICH–GCP and, in many countries, law).

Whatever their motivation, it is vital that potential subjects fully understand that there may be no direct benefit to themselves. It is important to ensure that, if they decide to participate, they have no misconceptions – they must be aware that they might receive a placebo rather than the active drug, and that they might not get the 'choice' of treatment they would have preferred (eg, surgery instead of a minimally invasive procedure).

Follow-up Visits

The hard work continues even after a subject has been enrolled into a study. In order to ensure that subjects make a useful contribution to the research, you must make sure that they feel comfortable taking part and, where possible, withdrawal before the end of the study should be avoided.

The process of retention starts in the recruitment phase. If a potential subject feels pressurized into entering the study or does not fully understand what participation involves, then he/she is more likely to become unhappy and withdraw.

The PI is responsible for ensuring that subjects are followed-up according to the study protocol, but often this is delegated to the CRC. In order to follow-up successfully, there are several aspects to consider:

- Choose subjects carefully (ie, consider whether the subject is likely to be reliable).
- Involve the family or friends of subjects in the process – understand who the subject listens to, and who they take advice from.
- Make sure that you or a colleague can be contacted and that you return calls from subjects.

Follow-up visits are an essential part of clinical research, but preparation is necessary to ensure they run smoothly:

- Ensure the PI is available if there are any queries to be resolved.
- When necessary, have a translator available and ensure that all study materials are translated into the languages required (these materials must be approved by the IRB/IEC).
- Send a reminder letter or phone the subject 2–3 weeks before the follow-up visit.
- Phone the subject between follow-up visits to maintain contact.
- Ensure that the subject remains happy regarding their involvement in the study and answer any questions at each follow-up visit.
- Ensure that all study-related procedures are completed at follow-up visits and that adverse event reporting is performed as specified in the protocol.

Some tips for ensuring a successful follow-up visit are listed in **Table 7**.

Subject Withdrawal

Although no one ever wants a subject to withdraw from a study, there will be times when this happens. It is the subject's right to withdraw at any time and without giving a reason. It is possible that the subject may decide to withdraw consent for all or part of the study. For example:

- Schedule appointments realistically, but do not rush subjects.
- Liaise with colleagues in other departments to ensure that appointment times can be met.
- Consider seeing subjects for follow-up out of normal working hours, if required.
- Consider transport issues, eg, car-parking facilities, bus times, and booking taxis for subjects. The informed consent process must make it clear whether subjects' traveling costs can be reimbursed.
- Make sure that subjects know how to contact you or another team member.
- If the site allows, have some light refreshments available, especially if fasting blood samples must be taken.
- Be sure to establish several possible channels of contact for the subject (eg, family or a friend at a different address).
- Reconfirm appointments close to the booked date.

Table 7. A survival guide to follow-up visits.

- The subject will not take the study medication, but is prepared to continue with follow-up visits and/or procedures. Most protocols will define how data from such subjects should be analyzed.
- The subject does not wish to undergo follow-up tests (eg, an angiogram), but is prepared to continue all other follow-up procedures, which may or may not include continuing with the study medication.
- The subject wants no further contact whatsoever, and no further data can be obtained from the subject. In some instances the subject might consent to allow the CRC to obtain survival data from his/her general physician or the national statistics office.

If a subject does withdraw from a study, their safety must always be considered and any standard care must be carried out as usual.

Conclusion

Subject recruitment and retention are necessary for a study to work. The points noted in this chapter will help you to effectively manage both recruitment and retention. This will help you to be a part of a successful study that provides an answer to an important clinical question, thereby changing practice for the benefit of people in the future.

References

1. Gamache V. Minimizing volunteer dropout. CenterWatch Monthly 2002;December:9-12.

2 Kermani F. Japanese R&D: branching out. Applied Clinical Trials 2004;August. Available from: www.actmagazine.com/ appliedclinicaltrials/article/articleDetail.jsp?id=1 09174. Accessed February 10, 2005.

3. Spilker B, Cramer J. Patient Recruitment in Clinical Trials. Philadelphia, PA: Lippincott-Raven Publishers, 1996.

4. Beasley D. Perfect harmony. Applied Clinical Trials 2004;November. Available from: www.actmagazine.com/appliedclinicaltrials/artic le/articleDetail.jsp?id=129272. Accessed February 10, 2005.

5. Cavalieri RJ. Effective advertising strategies for clinical research sites. Clinical Researcher 2003;3(5):12-17.

6. Goggin MJ. Introduction to the Work of Research Ethics Committees, 2nd Edition. London: The Association of the British Pharmaceutical Industry. Available from: www.abpi.org.uk/ publications/pdfs/Intro_research_ethics.pdf.

7. FDA Information Sheets. Guidance for Institutional Review Boards and Clinical Investigators: Recruiting Study Subjects. Update. Food and Drug Administration, 1998. Available from: www.fda.gov/oc/ohrt/irbs /toc4.html. Accessed February 10, 2005.

8. Neuer A. Treating study volunteers as customers. CenterWatch Monthly 2003;March:1-7.

9. Holt E. The HIPAA Privacy Rule, research, and IRBs. Applied Clinical Trials 2003;June. Available from:www.actmagazine.com/appliedclinicaltrials /article/articleDetail.jsp?id=80209. Accessed February 10, 2005.

10. Glover RL. The HIPAA Privacy Rule affects subject recruitment. Applied Clinical Trials 2002;November. Available from: www.actmagazine.com/appliedclinicaltrials/ article/articleDetail.jsp?id=82494. Accessed February 10, 2005.

11. EU Clinical Trial Directive. Available from: www.europa.eu.int/eur-lex/en/search/ search_lif.html. Accessed February 10, 2005.

Chapter 9

Documentation

Paula Jones-Wright

Introduction

This chapter provides an overview of the documentation process in clinical trials, including the definitions of documentation related to the International Conference on Harmonisation guidelines for Good Clinical Practice (ICH–GCP). As discussed in **Chapter 2**, ICH–GCP is an international standard for the design, conduct, performance, monitoring, auditing, recording, analysis, and reporting of clinical trials. Several countries have incorporated parts of ICH–GCP into their national law, while others recommend, but do not legally enforce, compliance with ICH–GCP.

Following ICH–GCP provides assurance that the data and reported results from a clinical research study are credible and accurate, and that the rights, integrity, and confidentiality of trial subjects are protected. This is achieved by recording, handling, and storing all clinical trial information in a way that allows it to be accurately reported, interpreted, and verified [1]. Through a precise data collection process, you, the clinical research coordinator (CRC), can ensure that the clinical trial results reported are accurate, thereby preserving research integrity and human subjects protection. If any inaccuracies are introduced into the data collection process then the results will be invalidated, and the participants will have been subjected to risk for no reason.

This chapter explains the terminology and principles behind accurate data collection and record keeping, confidentiality, documenting and reporting adverse events (AEs), quality assurance and quality control of data, audits, and document retention, and gives practical advice on how to deal with these issues on a day-to-day basis.

Definitions

Before further aspects of data collection are discussed, it is useful to review the definitions of some commonly used terms. All have a specific ICH–GCP definition.

Documentation

According to ICH–GCP, documentation is defined as "all records, in any form... that describe or record the methods, conduct, and/or results of a trial, the factors affecting a trial, and the actions taken" [1]. As a crucial part of your ongoing responsibilities, you will be involved in the documentation of all the events that take place in the clinical trial on a daily basis. The US Food and Drug Administration (FDA)'s viewpoint regarding documentation is that "if it was not documented then it was not done". An example of an important document is the informed consent form, which the subject signs prior to enrollment into a study.

Source Documents

Source documents are the original documents, data, and records collected in a trial. Examples of source documents include "hospital records, clinic and office charts, laboratory notes, memoranda, subjects' diaries or evaluation checklists, pharmacy dispensing records, recorded data from automated instruments, copies or transcriptions certified after verification as being accurate copies, microfiches, photographic negatives, microfilm or magnetic media, X-rays, subject files, and records kept at the pharmacy, at the laboratories and at medico-technical departments involved in the clinical trial" [1]. Source documents are a type of essential document, discussed in the next paragraph.

Essential Documents

The documents that "individually and collectively permit evaluation of the conduct of a trial and the quality of the data produced" are called the essential documents for the conduct of a clinical trial [1].

It is important to note the difference between source documents and essential documents: essential documents include additional documents beyond those considered to be source documents, eg, the investigator's brochure, the protocol, and the contract. The essential documents required by ICH-GCP are outlined in section 8 of the guidance [1].

Source Data

The source data are "all information in the original records and certified copies of original records of clinical findings, observations, or other activities in a clinical trial necessary for the reconstruction and evaluation of the trial. Source data are contained in source documents (original records or certified copies)" [1]. Certified copies are usually those where the source documents have been stamped with a recognized or certified hospital or clinic logo, which is used to validate hospital and site documentation.

Case Report Forms

Source data must be recorded onto the case report form (CRF) provided by the sponsor. The CRF is "a printed, optical [ie, one that can be read or viewed clearly], or electronic document designed to record all of the protocol required information to be reported to the sponsor on each trial subject" [1]. CRFs record the data that are required as outlined by the procedures in the protocol.

You will receive a binder containing CRFs for each research subject. CRCs typically spend a considerable amount of time transcribing data from the original records or source documents to CRFs. At some sites, the actual transcription process is done by a research assistant. More often, CRFs are printed on no-carbon-required paper that allows for duplicate copies to be dispersed between the sponsor and the research site.

Preparation and Filing

The process of completing and filing the essential documents for a clinical trial begins before the first subject is enrolled into the study. The process starts with the signing of a confidentiality agreement, which is sent to the investigator by the sponsor and is then signed by the investigator and returned to the sponsor. This agreement testifies that the site will keep the sponsor's proprietary information regarding the clinical trial confidential. Other examples of prestudy documents are the contract, forms required by regulatory bodies prior to study start up, the budget, and other forms depending on the sponsor's requests and requirements.

All trial documents must be filed systematically at the site. Proper organization of regulatory documents and study files will keep the study within a controlled environment and will help to improve regulatory compliance during the trial. It is

Document group	Examples
Regulatory documents	US Food and Drug Administration Form 1572, new drug application
Study documents	Case report forms, randomization codes
Human subject records	Results of clinical tests, informed consent forms
Correspondence with the institutional review board/ independent ethics committee	Reports of adverse events, regulatory approval documents
Correspondence with the sponsor	Letters arranging site monitoring visits, correspondence relating to adverse events
General information	Investigator's brochure, CVs/résumés of site staff
Regulatory references	International Conference on Harmonisation guidelines for Good Clinical Practice, Declaration of Helsinki, Belmont Report

Table 1. A guide to useful document groups for filing.

the investigator's responsibility to maintain the study files, although this responsibility will often be delegated to you during the study. You should begin to prepare the study files at the initiation of the clinical trial.

When preparing the files, you should develop a single, organized method to ensure consistency in the filing process and develop a system that allows for the rapid retrieval of documents and files. This filing system can be formalized in the site's standard operating procedures (SOPs). The document groups in **Table 1** can be used to create a filing system.

A regulatory binder that includes all pertinent information should be created and kept up-to-date [2]. A checklist of the information to be included is given in **Table 2**.

Data Collection

Data collection involves working as a team member with the study monitor (also known as the clinical research associate) employed by the sponsor, at all monitoring visits, to ensure that the documents are accurate, properly completed, and filed correctly. You should also communicate in an ongoing fashion with the institutional review board (IRB)/independent ethics committe (IEC) regarding the documentation and records for the clinical trial. In the USA, it is common practice

---

The regulatory binder should include:

- signed contract
- budget
- confidentiality agreement
- CVs/résumés of the investigator and clinical research coordinator
- signed protocol and amendments
- insurance statement (if applicable)
- normal laboratory ranges
- investigator brochure
- protocol
- institutional review board/research ethics board approval

Table 2. Regulatory binder checklist.

for CRCs to review study records with the IRB/IEC before the sponsor or the FDA carries out a monitoring visit.

At each subject visit, you will conduct specific trial-related tests and procedures, such as interviews and physical assessments, while recording information on the source documents. Subjects are also sometimes asked to record data in diaries, which are taken home with them and brought back on subsequent clinic visits. The data contained within subject diaries often pertain to quality-of-life questions or medication compliance.

Research data that are collected by the investigator or other staff, such as the results of physical examinations, are usually transcribed from the source documents to CRFs by the CRC. You will also transcribe any information recorded by the subjects themselves (ie, from their diaries) to CRFs.

The source documents used to collect the specific information necessary for the clinical trial – which is then recorded onto CRFs – are often developed by the CRC. They should be designed to accurately collect the required information in an organized manner. In most source documents, the information and checklists used will reflect the information required on the CRF. It is also imperative that transcribed data are validated and carefully proofed to avoid transcription errors. This is part of the quality control process, which is covered later in this chapter (see p.134).

It is vital that you create an organized system for maintaining clinical trial source documents and CRFs, while at the same time protecting the confidentiality of participant records. Sponsors sometimes provide a checklist of visit procedures that can be useful for helping you to track the completion of required assessments. If a checklist is not provided by the sponsor then source documents that reflect the data that need to be collected for the clinical trial can help with tracking. A checklist of visit procedures may also be given in the site's SOPs (if available).

Confidentiality and Access to Documentation

In order for you to collect data during the clinical trial process, direct access to patient information is required. You will facilitate this access. The site will give the sponsor direct access to patient information, in compliance with Good Clinical Practice (GCP) responsibilities and as defined in the contract with the sponsor. You will ensure this direct access by obtaining the subject's signature on the informed consent document. The informed consent document should state that direct access is an essential element of the trial in order to examine, analyze, verify, and reproduce any records and reports needed for the evaluation of trial results [1].

During the informed consent process, you must also inform subjects that direct access to their personal/protected health information (PHI) will be necessary as part of their participation in the research. In granting this permission to the sponsor, you must verify patient permission according to local privacy laws, such as the Health Insurance Portability and Accountability Act (HIPAA) in the USA, Directive 95/46/EC in the European Union, and the Personal Information Protection and Electronic Documents Act in Canada (see **Chapter 2**). All parties that come into contact with subjects' identities and the sponsor's proprietary information – be they domestic or foreign regulatory authorities, the sponsor's monitors, CRCs, investigators, institutional officials, or auditors – should take all reasonable precautions to maintain confidentiality of the data [1].

Documenting Adverse Events

According to ICH–GCP, "Before a trial is initiated, foreseeable risks and inconveniences should be weighed against the anticipated benefit for the individual trial subject and society. A trial should be initiated and continued only if the anticipated benefits justify the risks" [1].

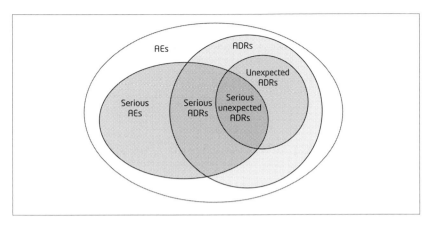

Figure 1. The relationship between adverse events (AEs) and adverse drug reactions (ADRs).

You must comply with GCP in order to provide public assurance that the rights, safety, and wellbeing of subjects are protected. AE and serious adverse event (SAE) reporting enforces this commitment to subject safety and ensures the development of drugs that are efficacious and safe. In fact, you should inform subjects of any potential AEs or SAEs as part of the ongoing informed consent process.

Definitions

Before discussing safety reporting, it is important to define the key terms, several of which have specific ICH–GCP definitions. These terms are described in the following paragraphs; the relationship between them is shown in **Figure 1**, while an example of how to classify a reaction is given in **Figure 2**.

Adverse Event

ICH–GCP states that an AE is: "Any untoward medical occurrence in a patient or clinical investigation subject administered a pharmaceutical product and which does not necessarily have a causal relationship with this treatment. An AE can therefore be any unfavorable and unintended sign (including an abnormal laboratory finding), symptom, or disease temporally associated with the use of a medicinal (investigational) product, whether or not related to the medicinal (investigational) product" [1].

An AE can be unrelated, possibly related, or definitely related to the treatment. An AE can also be expected (ie, as outlined in the investigator's brochure) or unexpected (ie, not identified by preclinical or earlier phases of the research conducted on the investigational product).

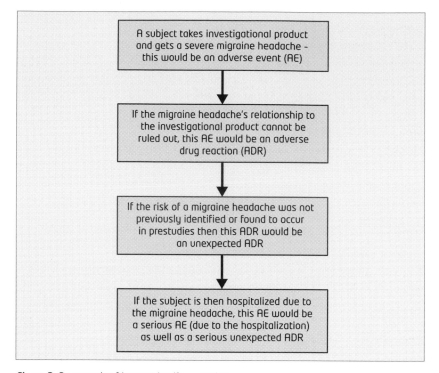

Figure 2. An example of how to classify a reaction.

Adverse Drug Reaction

The ICH–GCP definition of an adverse drug reaction (ADR) is very comprehensive. It states: "In the preapproval clinical experience with a new medicinal product or its new usages, particularly as the therapeutic dose(s) may not be established: all noxious and unintended responses to a medicinal product related to any dose should be considered adverse drug reactions. The phrase 'responses to a medicinal product' means that a causal relationship between a medicinal product and an adverse event is at least a reasonable possibility, ie, the relationship cannot be ruled out. Regarding marketed medicinal products: a response to a drug which is noxious and unintended and which occurs at doses normally used in man for prophylaxis, diagnosis, or therapy of diseases or for modification of physiological function" [1].

ADRs are a type of AE, although not all AEs are ADRs. This is because an AE does not necessarily have a causal relationship with the treatment, whereas an ADR has at least a reasonable possibility of being related to the treatment.

Unexpected Adverse Drug Reaction

ICH–GCP defines an unexpected ADR as: "An adverse reaction, the nature or severity of which is not consistent with the applicable product information (eg, investigator's brochure for an unapproved investigational product or package insert/summary of product characteristics for an approved product)." [1].

Serious Adverse Event

An SAE is: "Any untoward medical occurrence that at any dose: results in death, is life threatening, requires inpatient hospitalization or prolongation of existing hospitalization, results in persistent or significant disability/incapacity, or is a congenital anomaly/birth defect" [1]. An ADR can be, or can become, an SAE, eg, a subject may have an ADR and be hospitalized.

Serious Unexpected Adverse Drug Reaction

A serious unexpected ADR is an SAE that is not identified in nature, severity, or frequency in the risk information set out in the investigator's brochure, the informed consent form, or on the label of the drug.

Causality Assessment

A causality assessment is the process by which it is determined whether there is a reasonable possibility that the investigational drug caused or contributed to the AE. It includes assessing temporal relationships, dechallenge/rechallenge information, association (or lack of association) with underlying disease, and the presence (or absence) of a more likely cause [2,3].

Clinical Significance

Clinical significance describes a change in a subject's clinical condition that is regarded as important, whether or not it is due to the treatment (investigational product). Some statistically significant changes (eg, in blood test results) have no clinical significance. The criterion or criteria for clinical significance should be stated in the protocol [2,3].

Risk

Risk is defined in clinical trials as the probability of harm or discomfort affecting subjects. The level of acceptable risk will vary depending on the condition for which a product is being tested. For example, a treatment for sore throats will be expected to have a low incidence of side effects. However, unpleasant side effects might be an acceptable risk when testing a promising treatment for a life-threatening illness [3].

- Route, dose, date, and time of administration of the investigational product
- Date of report to sponsor
- Nature of AE or SAE
- Date and time of onset of AE or SAE
- Duration
- Resolution (if applicable)
- Laboratory data
- Concomitant medications
- Investigator's assessment of severity classification
- Investigator's assessment of the relationship to the investigational product
- The details of the person reporting the AE or SAE
- Actions that were taken
- Follow-up information

Table 3. Information usually requested by sponsors regarding adverse events (AEs) and serious adverse events (SAEs) [4].

Safety

Safety is relative freedom from harm. In clinical trials, this refers to an absence of harmful side effects resulting from use of the investigational product. It can be assessed by laboratory testing of biological samples, special tests and procedures, psychiatric evaluation, and/or physical examination of subjects [3].

Reporting

You should record all AEs and SAEs in the source documents and on the CRFs provided by the sponsor. The ICH–GCP guidelines have resulted in the standardization of these reporting processes by CRCs and, for each trial, the sponsor will outline in detail their own additional procedures for reporting and recording AEs and SAEs [4,5]. You should also be aware of the reporting requirements of the local IRB/IEC.

You should keep concise records of the IRB/IEC reporting process. You must report all SAEs and unexpected AEs immediately, or within 24 hours of being informed about the event, by telephone and/or fax to the sponsor according to the sponsor's SOPs. Following this, most sponsors will require a written report detailing the event to be submitted to them within 5 days. The sponsor will outline the specific reporting procedures in the protocol. The information that must be provided is outlined in **Table 3**.

Suspected connection between AE and investigational product	Definition
No relationship	The AE is not associated with use of the investigational product
Remote relationship	The AE is remotely associated with use of the investigational product
Possible relationship	The AE has a causal relationship with use of the investigational product and follows a sequence from the administration of the investigational product. However, the AE could have also been produced by the subject's medical condition or other therapies
Probable relationship	The AE has a causal relationship with use of the investigational product and follows a sequence from the administration of the investigational product and stops once the investigational product is discontinued. The AE cannot be explained by the subject's medical condition or clinical state
Highly probable relationship	The AE has a causal relationship with use of the investigational product and follows a sequence from the administration of the investigational product and stops once the investigational product is discontinued. The AE is confirmed by recurrence of the AE with repeat exposure to the investigational product

Table 4. Commonly used categories to define the relationship between an adverse event (AE) and an investigational product [3].

All information about AEs or SAEs should be reported in the CRFs supplied by the sponsor. This data will then be validated by the monitor, who will check that the data recorded in the CRFs correlates with the information documented in the source documents.

In addition to capturing the required information for AEs and SAEs, you should also complete the required sponsor documentation (eg, the MedWatch form in the USA [6]). The investigator should determine the extent of the relationship between the AE and the investigational product using the categories in **Table 4** – these categories are used by most sponsors.

Classification

AEs in which a relationship to the investigational product cannot be ruled out, whether expected (ie, as outlined in the investigator's brochure) or unexpected (ie, not identified by preclinical or earlier phases of the research conducted on the investigational product), should be recorded as ADRs. The investigator should assess the severity of the AE using the sponsor's definitions, or by using the following criteria [3]:

- Mild – the AE resolves without treatment.
- Moderate – the AE resolves or is tolerated with specific treatment, without affecting the activities of the clinical trial.
- Severe – the AE does not resolve or is not tolerated with treatment.

The classification of the severity of AEs and SAEs, and the assessment of the relationship to the investigational product, should only be made by the investigator: this is a medical decision that only an investigator can make. Usually, the investigator is a licensed physician, although, more rarely, they could be a pharmacist or other research professional (this requirement varies according to country – in Canada, for example, investigators must be a licensed physician). If the AE or SAE results in the investigator breaking the randomization code, you must document what happened at the time of the event in the source documents and inform the sponsor of the reason for the code being broken.

Quality Assurance and Quality Control

Since there are many documentation requirements that you must be aware of in order to help run a clinical trial smoothly, it is extremely important that everything is documented accurately, completely, legibly, and in a timely fashion. Problems will begin as soon as anything is not kept up-to-date. Monitors will help you to promptly identify any problems, but, if these are not rectified quickly, and if a good system is not in place, it will be very difficult to produce all the data that the sponsor requires and almost impossible to pass a regulatory audit.

Ultimately, any inadequacies in documentation can increase risks to the research participants. To ensure the integrity of the trial data, a system of quality assurance (QA) and quality control (QC) should be used.

Responsibilities

According to ICH–GCP, "The sponsor is responsible for implementing and maintaining quality assurance and quality control systems with written SOPs to ensure that trials are conducted and data are generated, documented (recorded), and reported in compliance with the protocol, GCP, and the applicable country regulatory requirement(s)...

"Quality control should be applied to each stage of data handling to ensure that all data are reliable and have been processed correctly" [1].

This will assist in creating the appropriate documentation. The audit trail is documentation that allows for the total reconstruction of the course of events taking place during the implementation of the clinical trial protocol at the site [1]. This documentation is crucial at the time of an audit or inspection at the site, because it is the paper trail that will be reviewed by the inspection team. As the CRC, you are responsible for data integrity, which ensures that subject participation was maximized for generalizable knowledge.

Quality Assurance
According to ICH–GCP, QA involves: "All those planned and systematic actions that are established to ensure that the trial is performed and the data are generated, documented (recorded), and reported in compliance with GCP and the applicable country regulatory requirement(s)" [1]. A practical example of a QA process is the implementation of SOPs at a site.

Quality Control
QC is defined by ICH–GCP as: "The operational techniques and activities undertaken within the quality assurance system to verify that the requirements for quality of the trial-related activities have been fulfilled" [1]. The activities that are carried out at the site in the process of following the site's SOPs are an example of a QC process.

Data Verification
The process of data verification is completed by the monitor during the site visit. This process involves validating the data or information that you have recorded on the CRFs by comparing the CRFs with the source documents. ICH–GCP outlines the process of data validation in the responsibilities of sponsors and monitors; more specifically, "Monitoring is the act of overseeing the progress of a clinical trial, and of ensuring that it is conducted, recorded, and reported in accordance with the protocol, Standard Operating Procedures (SOPs), Good Clinical Practice (GCP), and the applicable regulatory requirement(s)" [1].

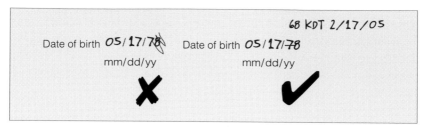

Figure 3. How to make a data change.

According to ICH–GCP, the purposes of trial monitoring are to verify that [1]:

- the rights and wellbeing of human subjects are protected
- trial data are accurate, complete, and verifiable from source documents
- the trial is conducted in compliance with the currently approved protocol/amendment(s), GCP, and applicable regulatory requirement(s)

It is the sponsor's responsibility to ensure that clinical trials are adequately monitored. The sponsor should determine the appropriate extent and nature of monitoring and notify you of this. The monitor will act as the main line of communication between the sponsor and the investigator/CRC.

The monitor should submit a written report to the sponsor after each site visit or trial-related communication. The monitoring report is defined by ICH–GCP as, "A written report from the monitor to the sponsor after each site visit and/or other trial-related communication according to the sponsor's SOPs" [1]. Reports should include a summary of what the monitor has reviewed and statements concerning the significant findings/facts, deviations and deficiencies, conclusions, actions taken or to be taken, and/or actions recommended to secure compliance.

Corrections and Amendments

ICH–GCP suggests that the sponsor should provide you with guidance about making data corrections, and you should retain records of all data changes and corrections [1]. When you makes changes or corrections to a CRF or source document, the changes should be dated, initialed, and explained (if necessary), and the original entry should not be obscured in any way (see **Figure 3**). This applies to both written and electronic changes or corrections.

Most electronic data capture (EDC) systems have a process to change data electronically. Should an EDC system be in place, you should request training on the entire system: this is often done at the investigators' meeting prior to the start of the study.

Regulatory Audits/Inspections

It is essential to develop an audit trail through accurate documentation of the course of events taking place during the study. Not only does this demonstrate proof of compliance with guidelines and regulations, but, in the case of an audit or inspection, this audit trail allows for the reconstruction of all clinical study procedures.

During an audit, the audit team will conduct a systematic and independent examination of study-related activities and documents to determine whether the evaluated trial-related activities were conducted, and the data were recorded, analyzed, and accurately reported according to the protocol, sponsor's/site's SOPs, GCP, and the applicable country and state or local regulations and/or guidelines [1].

During an audit you should be available, in addition to the investigator, to answer any questions that the audit team might have. You should also organize a room for the audit team and the study documents that will need to be reviewed during the audit process.

CRF Data Review, Clarification, and Resolution, and Handling Data Queries

The monitor will collect data from the site by retrieving CRF copies at site visits. Most CRFs are now composed of paper that allows three copies to be made at once – the top copy is retrieved by the sponsor, while the other carbon copies stay at the site. Once the sponsor obtains the data, a special data clarification and resolution system is used to verify the accuracy (including subject eligibility and overall quality) of the data. Each CRF collected will be reviewed for the following:

- subject eligibility
- subject evaluability

- AEs
- SAEs
- any other significant findings
- completeness
- signature authorization

The data are then entered into a database at the sponsor's site and data clarification forms (DCFs) will be generated for the statistical and clinical trial reports. Any data that are ambiguous or illegible will result in the sponsor sending a data query to the site in the form of a DCF. You must then clarify the data query at, or prior to, the next monitoring visit. All changes you make to the CRFs in response to a query should be recorded on the DCF – this form becomes an extension of the CRF. You should only make corrections to CRFs that can be validated by the protocol procedures.

You should not change data at the request of the monitor if there is disagreement concerning the clinical significance of the data (eg, causality statements for AEs or SAEs). You must always discuss these discrepancies with the investigator, who will give his/her final interpretation. You should also ask the investigator to sign all DCFs in order to approve all data clarifications [2]. This should be done after the date of the last entry to verify that the investigator is aware of all of the changes.

Document Retention

In the same way that all clinical research documentation must be properly filed and maintained, measures must be taken to prevent the accidental or premature destruction of clinical trial documents. Institutions and sponsors should develop and publish a record retention policy, and ICH–GCP states that it is the responsibility of the sponsor to inform the investigator and the CRC as to when essential documents no longer need to be retained [1]. You should take responsibility for ensuring that these document retention policies are followed.

Most retention policies are based on ICH–GCP recommendations, which state: "Sponsor-specific essential documents should be retained until at least 2 years after the last approval of a marketing application in an ICH region and until there are no pending or contemplated marketing applications in an ICH region or at least

2 years have elapsed since the formal discontinuation of clinical development of the investigational product" [1]. Most sponsors in the USA and Europe require 15 years' record retention; in Canada, the regulations mandate 25 years' record retention [7].

Requirements for record retention vary with the type of research conducted and provisions of the investigator's funding source. It is highly recommended that investigators and CRCs clearly understand the retention requirements of their sponsor.

The Department of Health and Human Services (HHS) and the FDA have regulations related to retention of protocol records. The HHS regulation (45 CFR 46.115) provides direction for all research conducted or supported by any federal department or agency. This regulation states that IRB records relating to research conducted shall be retained for at least 3 years after completion of the research. The FDA regulation (21 CFR 56.115) is virtually identical; it also states that IRB records must be retained for at least 3 years after completion of the research.

Clinical trials with an FDA investigational new drug application must additionally comply with 21 CFR 312.57 and 21 CFR 312.62. These regulations apply to investigational drug records, investigator financial interest records, and patient case histories. Both regulations require that the sponsor retain records and reports for 2 years after a marketing application is approved for the drug. If an application is not approved for the drug, the sponsor retains records and reports until 2 years after shipment and delivery of the drug for investigational use is discontinued, and the FDA has been so notified.

Investigators and research sites are encouraged to maintain research records for longer periods, if practicable. Requirements for record retention vary with the type of research conducted and provisions of the investigator's funding source. It is highly recommended that investigators and CRCs clearly understand the retention requirements of their sponsor and their institution/research site.

Conclusion

Filing systems and documentation maintenance processes are important in conducting any type of clinical research. Keeping accurate source documents as well as source data is an essential component of your job. The process of data transfer from source documents to CRFs is critical for the success of the clinical trial, and so QA and QC are vital for data validation. Accurate and timely AE and SAE reporting is essential for the protection of study participants, and good documentation of the process is key. Good study documentation is also important for the accurate reconstruction of the clinical trial process. This is a scientific requirement, as well as being crucial for an audit or inspection.

Compliance with international guidelines and national regulations will help to ensure that the process of recording, handling, and storing clinical trial information is done in a way that allows it to be accurately reported, interpreted, and verified. Through a precise data collection process, you can ensure that the clinical trial results are accurate.

References

1. International Conference on Harmonisation of Technical Requirements for Registration of Pharmaceuticals for Human Use. ICH Harmonised Tripartite Guideline: Guideline for Good Clinical Practice. E6. Available from: www.ich.org. Accessed November 17, 2004.

2. Paula Jones-Wright, ClinCoach Inc. Standard Operating Procedures for Clinical Research Sites, 2005.

3. Spilker B. Guide to Clinical Trials. New York, NY: Lippincott Williams & Wilkins, 1991.

4. Fedor C, Grosbard A. The Coordinators' Forum Part 10: Adverse event recording and reporting - protecting human research participants' safety. Clinical Researcher 2003;3(3):22-4.

5. Fedor, C. The Coordinators' Forum. Follow-up to adverse event recording and reporting. Clinical Researcher 2003;3(5):18-20.

6. FDA Form 3500A - Mandatory Reporting. Available from: www.fda.gov/medwatch/SAFETY/3500A.pdf. Accessed Februrary 17, 2005.

7. Dench A, Rammell E, Vaillant S. Retention of clinical trial record, medical records and essential document. Clinical Researcher 2002;2(8):24-8.

Chapter 10

Assuring Quality in Clinical Trials: Monitoring, Audits, and Inspections

Paula Jones-Wright

"Good Clinical Practice [GCP] is an international ethical and scientific quality standard for designing, conducting, recording, and reporting trials..." [1].

Introduction

Quality in clinical trials is essential, and all parties involved in the conduct of a clinical trial bear responsibility for either assuring or ensuring quality. There are many people/groups involved in the regulation and quality of clinical trials, and these are listed in **Table 1**.

This chapter provides an overview of quality measures, focusing specifically on monitoring, audits, and inspections. Specific activities related to ensuring quality at study close-out are also described. Clearly, not all trials are sponsored, and hence not all trials are subject to external monitoring. However, the responsibility of the principal investigator (PI) and study team to maintain quality remains. An understanding of the role of monitoring, audits, and inspections in clinical trials should enable you, the clinical research coordinator (CRC), to maintain the highest possible standards of quality.

Person/group	Means of ensuring/assuring quality
Principal investigator and study team, including clinical research coordinator Local regulations	Protocol compliance Standard processes
Sponsor Audits Standard operating procedures	On-site monitoring
Regulatory authorities	Inspections
Data protection agencies	Inspections
Institutional review board/ independent ethics committee	Continuing review

Table 1. Partners in quality.

"The act of overseeing the progress of a clinical trial, and of ensuring that it is conducted, recorded, and reported in accordance with the protocol, standard operating procedures, Good Clinical Practice... and the applicable regulatory requirement(s)."

Table 2. The International Conference on Hamonisation guidelines for Good Clinical Practice definition of monitoring [1].

Monitoring

Monitoring is carried out by a monitor (also known as the clinical research associate [CRA]) on behalf of the sponsor of a trial, and is the process of ensuring that the site is conducting the trial in accordance with the protocol, the sponsor's standard operating procedures (SOPs), GCP, and applicable local regulatory requirements (see **Table 2**). Monitoring will enable you to check that you are conducting the trial correctly, and will give you the opportunity to identify any problems that might impact the validity of the trial.

The Monitor

You should remember that the monitor is a professional. Monitors receive extensive training and are required to be clinical trial experts. The monitor should be thoroughly familiar with the investigational product(s), the protocol, the written informed consent form and any other written information to be provided to subjects, the sponsor's SOPs, GCP, and applicable local regulatory requirement(s) [1].

Before the trial the monitor can help with:	Communication with the sponsor
	Practical advice and support
	Study team training
	Advice on site and study management
During the trial the monitor will review:	Source document verification
	Adverse event reporting
	Subject recruitment
	Record management
After the trial the monitor will review:	Investigational product accountability (eg, ensuring destruction/return to sponsor)
	Archiving
	Study close-out activities

Table 3. What does the monitor do?

Monitors generally have a wealth of experience of clinical trial conduct and should be considered as a valuable resource by the study team. Establishing a good rapport with the monitor should be one of your key aims, as this will both facilitate communication with the sponsor and improve the efficiency with which the clinical trial is run at your site.

Monitors have important responsibilities before, during, and after a trial, and you should seek their advice as early as possible in order to help get your site up to speed for a trial. The key responsibilities of the monitor at different stages of a trial are summarized in **Table 3**.

Study Monitoring Visits

Monitoring is the act of overseeing the progress of a clinical trial, and of ensuring that the trial is conducted, recorded, and reported in accordance with the protocol, SOPs, GCP, and applicable local regulatory requirement(s) [1]. Monitoring of clinical trials has many purposes and, as discussed in the International Conference on Harmonisation guidelines for Good Clinical Practice (ICH–GCP) [1], monitoring visits verify that:

- the rights and wellbeing of human subjects are protected
- the reported trial data are accurate, complete, and verifiable from source documents
- the conduct of the trial is in compliance with the current, approved protocol/amendment(s), GCP, and applicable local regulatory requirement(s)

According to ICH–GCP, it is the sponsor's responsibility to guarantee that trials are adequately monitored [1]. The sponsor and monitor will determine the appropriate extent and nature of monitoring, and this decision will be based on many factors – including the number of participants enrolled in the study, the number of data discrepancies at the site, and the experience level at the site. This determination will also be based on the study's objectives, purpose, design (including whether it is blinded), complexity, and endpoints.

To enable the monitor to ensure that the trial is conducted appropriately and in accordance with GCP, there is a need for on-site monitoring before, during, and after the clinical trial, along with investigator training and meetings, and extensive written guidance [1]. As a CRC, you should understand the appropriate frequency, extent, and nature of monitoring.

The Monitor's Responsibilities

To ensure that the study is conducted and documented properly, the monitor carries out the following 17 activities at the site (as listed in ICH–GCP) according to the sponsor's requirements and SOPs [1].

1. The monitor acts as the main line of communication between the sponsor, PI, and CRC.

2. The monitor verifies that the PI and CRC have:

   - adequate qualifications
   - resources that will remain adequate throughout the clinical trial period
   - facilities to safely and properly conduct the clinical trial (including laboratories, equipment, and staff) that are, and will remain, adequate throughout the clinical trial period

3. The monitor verifies that, for the investigational product(s):

   - storage times and conditions are acceptable, and that supplies are sufficient
   - it is supplied only to participants who are eligible to receive it and at the dose(s) specified in the protocol

- participants are provided with necessary instructions on how to properly use, handle, store, and return it
- its receipt, use, and return at the site are controlled and documented adequately
- the disposal of unused investigational product(s) at the trial site complies with the regulatory requirement(s) applicable in that country and with the sponsor's instructions

4. The monitor verifies that the PI follows the approved protocol and all approved amendment(s), if any.

5. The monitor verifies that written informed consent has been obtained before each participant enters the clinical trial.

6. The monitor ensures that the PI and CRC receive the current investigator's brochure, all documents, and all trial supplies needed to conduct the trial properly and to comply with the applicable regulatory requirement(s) in that country.

7. The monitor ensures that the PI, CRC, and trial staff are adequately informed about the trial.

8. The monitor verifies that the PI, CRC, and trial staff are performing the specified trial functions in accordance with the protocol and any other written agreement between the sponsor and the PI/institution, and have not delegated these functions to unauthorized individuals.

9. The monitor verifies that the PI is enrolling only eligible participants.

10. The monitor reports the participant recruitment rate.

11. The monitor verifies that source documents and other trial records are accurate, complete, kept up-to-date, and maintained.

12. The monitor verifies that the PI has provided all required reports, notifications, applications, and submissions, and that these documents are accurate, complete, timely, legible, dated, and identify the trial.

13. The monitor checks the accuracy and completeness of case report form (CRF) entries, source documents, and other trial-related records, verifying that:

- the data required by the protocol are reported accurately on the CRFs and are consistent with the source documents
- any modifications to dose and/or therapy are well documented for each of the trial subjects
- adverse events (AEs), concomitant medications, and concurrent illnesses are reported on the CRFs in accordance with the protocol
- visits that subjects have failed to make, tests that have not been conducted, and examinations that have not been performed are clearly reported as such on the CRFs
- all withdrawals and dropouts of participants enrolled in the trial are reported and explained on the CRFs

14. The monitor informs the PI and CRC of any CRF entry error, omission, or illegibility. The monitor should ensure that appropriate corrections, additions, or deletions are made, dated, explained (if necessary), and initialed by the PI or by an authorized member of the trial staff. This authorization should be documented.

15. The monitor determines whether all AEs have been reported appropriately within the time periods required by GCP, the protocol, the institutional review board (IRB)/independent ethics committee (IEC), the sponsor, and the applicable regulatory requirement(s) for that country.

16. The monitor determines whether the PI and CRC are maintaining the essential documents.

17. The monitor communicates deviations from the protocol, SOPs, GCP, and the applicable regulatory requirements to the PI/CRC and takes appropriate action designed to prevent recurrence of the detected deviations.

To enable the monitor to carry out their responsibilities, you should ensure that you and the site are ready for the monitoring visit (see **Table 4**).

> **Clinical research team members**
>
> Make sure that the study team is ready for the monitoring visit and that all team members required by the monitor will be present, eg, the investigator and clinical research coordinator.
>
> **Documents**
>
> Ensure that all documents required by the monitor are ready for review, ie, case report forms, source documents, etc.
>
> **Space**
>
> The monitor will require space and facilities in which to work and meet with members of the study team. Communicate with the monitor to find out how best you can meet these requirements.
>
> **Time**
>
> Allow for adequate time to meet with the monitor. Make sure that other members of the study team schedule time to answer any questions.

Table 4. Preparing for a monitoring visit.

The Monitoring Report

At every site visit, the monitor will produce an official account called a monitoring report. This written evaluation is transferred from the monitor to the sponsor after each site visit and will include all trial-related communications with the site staff, as specified in the sponsor's SOP requirements [1].

The monitor's report should include the date, site, his/her name, and the name of the PI and CRC (or any other individual[s] contacted during the site visit). A summary will be included of what the monitor reviewed, with statements concerning significant findings/facts, deviations and deficiencies, conclusions, actions taken or to be taken, and/or actions recommended by the monitor in order to guarantee GCP and compliance with the protocol [1]. Prior to the next visit, you should use the monitor's report as a checklist in order to clarify any information summarized in the report.

The Sponsor's Expectations of the CRC

The monitor acts as the central line of communication between you and the sponsor and, thus, the site. You need to enhance this communication by developing a positive working relationship with the monitor.

The sponsor will expect you to understand your general roles and responsibilities, as specified in ICH–GCP, and to be knowledgeable about clinical research. You will be expected to manage and coordinate the clinical trial – from the stage of prestudy

The sponsor will expect you to:

- follow Good Clinical Practice
- understand and follow the protocol and protocol amendments
- adhere to inclusion and exclusion criteria for enrolling eligible participants into the clinical trial
- use medical and nursing knowledge to recruit and screen participants
- become knowledgeable and resourceful about the disease being studied
- design and implement a recruitment strategy for the clinical trial
- be qualified in relation to the demands and requirements of the clinical trial
- recognize and assess limitations and seek assistance where needed
- produce an up-to-date CV/résumé
- have sufficient time to carry out the obligations and responsibilities of the research protocol
- know qualifications and limitations in relation to the protocol
- perform a self-learning needs assessment regarding the necessary skills required for the clinical trial
- become aware of safety issues regarding your own performance and the delegation of specific roles
- know the available resources to use to seek assistance with skills or other aspects of coordinating clinical trials
- become familiar with the preliminary data and scientific information regarding the clinical trial
- understand the investigator's brochure
- assess prestudy adverse events with the principal investigator for possible occurrence throughout the clinical trial
- provide other coordinators and clinical research staff with information to facilitate their understanding of the rationale for key features of the protocol
- assist with compliance with areas of the protocol (eg, dose, frequency/interval of administration, methods of administration, safety monitoring procedures for the investigational product)
- become aware of the most up-to-date guidelines and regulations in order to comply with, advocate, and follow them
- submit informed consent forms to the sponsor and IRB/IEC for approval
- document the entire process of informed consent
- follow the ethical principles of the "Declaration of Helsinki" and country-specific and local ethics guidelines to protect participants' rights
- follow local IRB/IEC standard operating procedures for informed consent
- be aware of the safety issues for the protocol and reporting procedures to the sponsor and IRB/IEC
- document all data and information accurately
- create and maintain study files and documents in an organized system
- use the ICH–GCP essential documents for the conduct of clinical trial research

Table 5. What will you be expected to do? ICH–GCP: International Conference on Harmonisation guidelines for Good Clinical Practice; IEC: independent ethics committee; IRB: institutional review board.

- organize work folders for every subject enrolled into the clinical trial
- complete case report forms in a neat and accurate fashion
- use appropriate source documentation for data sources and verification
- obtain and validate data information from original records of clinical findings and observations

Table 5. *Continued.*

feasibility assessment through to study close-out and completion – by using a plan of action [2]. A list of what will be expected of you is given in **Table 5**.

Data Verification

At every site visit, the monitor will verify that the data in the CRFs agree with the source documents. You should review the information in the clinical charts with the monitor and explain any discrepancies in the data. The monitor is looking for both accuracy and completeness of the data before taking them back to the sponsor for data processing [3].The monitor will conduct a general CRF check by examining the following:

- original assignment of the subject identification number
- ongoing accuracy in the recording of the subject identification number
- subject initials
- informed consent forms have been signed
- all data recorded in the CRF agree with the source documents

Each CRF will also be reviewed for the following:

- subject eligibility
- subject evaluability
- conduct of visits and procedures in compliance with the protocol
- AEs
- serious adverse events (SAEs)
- any other significant findings

Your responsibility for handling data queries extends to CRF data review, clarification, and resolution. Once the sponsor has obtained the data from the monitor, a special data clarification and resolution system is used to verify the accuracy of the data. Data are entered at the sponsor's site and data clarification

Before the study close-out monitoring visit you should:

- plan for the monitor's visit
- check that all requirements of the clinical trial agreement have been met
- conduct a thorough review of all documentation
- create an inventory of all documents
- inform the IRB/IEC of the trial's completion
- communicate with the study team about the trial's closure and seek their feedback
- notify the participant and his/her primary-care physician of the trial's closure
- ensure that all country-specific and ICH-GCP termination procedures have been followed
- check that the principal investigator has been advised by the sponsor of any potential health risks to participants

Table 6. Checklist of your responsibilities at study close-out. ICH-GCP International Conference on Harmonisation guidelines for Good Clinical Practice.

forms (DCFs) are generated for the statistical and clinical research reports. All data that are ambiguous or illegible will result in the generation of a data query by the sponsor. All changes made to CRFs should be recorded on a DCF, which becomes an extension of the CRF [3]. You should obtain DCFs from the monitor at each site visit. These will be produced on 'no carbon required' paper, and you will need to make appropriate corrections on them using the same procedures as for CRFs [3].

In order to minimize data queries you should obtain clear instructions from the monitor on the proper way to accurately collect the data and to ensure complete CRF information. In some situations, the sponsor will have an SOP manual for the completion of CRFs.

Procedures at the End of the Trial

At the end of the trial, a final study close-out visit by the monitor will take place and this will confirm the formal completion of the clinical trial. The procedures for study close-out should also be completed at the site if the sponsor, IRB/IEC, or PI discontinues the clinical trial. The closure of the clinical trial is a formal process that you, the CRC, should conduct, documenting all procedures in a final study report.

The CRC's responsibilities at study close-out are summarized in **Table 6**. The first stage in this process is to plan the date for the visit with the monitor and to request an agenda for the visit from the sponsor. You should ensure that all details in the clinical trial agreement/contract have been met (eg, payments to the site).

Documents

You should complete a thorough review of all clinical trial documents and ICH–GCP essential documents and review all files, such as the communications file, for the accuracy of the filing systems. You should review all outstanding items that were to be addressed from previous monitoring visits, and prepare for the possibility of a future inspection/audit by organizing all CRFs and study files [3].

You will need to complete a total inventory of all documents from study initiation to completion. All documents must be organized in chronological order and sequential versions. You should also resolve any discrepancies in the documents and ensure that all documents are correctly signed and dated. Any missing documents need to be found: if you are unable to locate these, you should explain this in a note to file [3].

Communication

You should also inform the IRB/IEC of the completion of the clinical trial and, once the final study report has been completed, this must also be submitted to the IRB/IEC. The format of this report will be indicated by the IRB/IEC's policies and procedures, and local site requirements.

It is crucial for you to communicate information about the study closure to all members of the clinical research team, and you should also notify appropriate departments of the close-out visit (eg, the pharmacy, laboratory, and X-ray department) [3]. It is important to obtain feedback from the research team members regarding their participation in the study so that you can communicate this information to the monitor at the final visit. You should also inform the staff about study results and any publications once these become available.

It is important that you notify participants of study completion as part of the ongoing informed consent process, and you should also notify participants' primary-care physicians. While doing this, you should ensure that the participant will receive proper medical care and treatment follow-up, especially if study completion means that the participant will no longer be receiving care directly from the PI. In addition, many CRCs notify subjects of the study results, when appropriate [3].

Close-out Procedures

When a study is discontinued by the PI, IRB/IEC, or regulatory bodies, you must follow the country-specific and ICH–GCP guidelines for termination procedures, especially regarding safety issues and reporting. You should check with the sponsor that all PIs involved in the study have been advised in writing of any potential risks to the health of clinical trial participants.

You should meet with the monitor to perform formal study close-out – all final data clarifications or data discrepancies should be resolved by reviewing all remaining DCFs for completeness [3]. If the final clinical study report is completed and available, you will need to arrange for the PI to sign this. The PI should discuss the publication of the final clinical study report with the sponsor's representative. You should initiate a discussion with the sponsor regarding feedback concerning your site's participation in the clinical trial. This feedback is important for maintaining an ongoing relationship with the sponsor for future studies and for improving/maintaining quality standards at your site [3].

Audits and Inspections

Sponsors and regulatory bodies carry out audits and inspections in order to implement quality assurance and to assess quality control processes at the site [1]. For example, in Canada the GCP Inspection Program of Health Canada conducts GCP inspections, while in the USA the US Food and Drug Administration (FDA) refers to the same process as an FDA audit, and the EU Clinical Trials Directive describes inspectors as being appointed by Member States to verify compliance with the provisions on Good Clinical Practice [4].

Audits/inspections differ from monitoring as they are concerned with compliance, eg, with ICH–GCP and the applicable local regulation(s), rather than the study's conduct. Audits/inspections are an opportunity for the sponsor or regulatory body to ensure that the quality of the trial is assured at that site.

You need to be prepared for both of these types of compliance monitoring, for all clinical trials being conducted at your site. When preparing for a sponsor's audit or inspection, you should find out its purpose and, if a regulatory body is involved, you should enquire as to the inspection's cause. The inspectors/auditors are usually experienced in GCP and will inspect for compliance with GCP.

> **Audit report**
>
> An evaluation of the results of an audit written by the sponsor's auditor.
>
> **Audit trail**
>
> Documentation that allows the course of events to be reconstructed.
>
> **Compliance**
>
> The state of conformity of a regulated party or a product with a legislative or regulatory requirement or a recognized standard.
>
> **Direct access**
>
> This refers to the permission to examine, analyze, verify, and reproduce records and reports that are important to the evaluation of a clinical trial. Any party (eg, domestic and foreign regulatory authorities, the sponsor's monitors and auditors) with direct access should take all reasonable precautions within the constraints of the applicable regulatory requirement(s) to maintain the confidentiality of subjects' identities and the sponsor's proprietary information.

Table 7. Useful definitions relating to Good Clinical Practice audits [1].

ICH–GCP defines an audit as: "A systematic and independent examination of trial-related activities and documents to determine whether trial-related activities were conducted, and the data were recorded, analyzed, and accurately reported according to the protocol, sponsor's SOPs, GCP, and the applicable regulatory requirement(s)" [1]. Some further definitions relating to GCP audits are given in **Table 7**.

For each audit, the inspector/auditor will have a formal plan and you should request information regarding the agenda for the audit prior to meeting the inspector/auditor at the site. Factors that will be considered include:

- the importance of the clinical trial submission to regulatory authorities
- the number of participants in the study
- the type and complexity of the study
- the level of risk to the participants (if any)

You should obtain a summary of the observations and findings of the auditor(s). The sponsor or auditor will usually provide an audit certificate along with their personal identification [1].

Preparing for an Audit/Inspection

It is crucial to prepare for an inspection from the onset of a clinical trial, and this is the most important aspect of study implementation that you will carry out. You should plan for potential audits/inspections by developing an audit/inspection action plan, including steps to take during an audit/inspection, and, prior to study initiation, you should also prepare for common problems that you will encounter.

If the site has existing SOPs, you should make sure that they are implemented fully and followed accurately. It is your responsibility to make available all requested clinical trial-related records for direct access, on request of the sponsor's monitor, the auditor, the IRB/IEC, or the regulatory authority(ies) [3].

Once you receive notification of an upcoming inspection/audit, you should ask the sponsor the following questions:

- What is the purpose of the audit/inspection?
- What is the plan for the audit?
- What audit/inspection procedures will be used?
- What format will audit/inspection reports take, and when will you receive them?
- When will follow-up after the audit/inspection take place and what format will this take?
- Will the site receive an audit certificate?
- What are the procedures for noncompliance?

You should then take the time to perform an internal audit to identify oversights, errors, and inaccuracies that may have occurred during the clinical trial. These should be resolved with accurate documentation on the course of events, including detailed explanations [3]. You should confirm that there is a complete and accurate audit trail of all documentation and ICH–GCP essential documents, and you should be prepared to demonstrate the accurate and safe conduct of the clinical trial according to ICH–GCP [3]. In an audit/inspection, it is also crucial to show compliance with the protocol, SOPs, ICH–GCP, and applicable regulatory requirements (eg, Health Canada Food and Drug Regulations [5], FDA regulations), and you must be able to demonstrate high standards of clinical research practice, medicine, science, and ethics [3].

You should be prepared to carry out a pre- and post-inspection interview. Topics for discussion might include:

- the relevant regulations, GCP guidelines, and site SOPs
- a review of the protocol
- the recruitment process
- the informed consent process
- the IRB/IEC review process

You will be expected to accompany the inspector on a tour of the facilities. Areas visited might include:

- clinics and examination rooms
- laboratories
- the pharmacy
- work areas for the study staff
- storage areas for the study drug and other study supplies

The audit process entails a comprehensive inspection of all aspects of research conduct and research procedures (see **Table 8**). An exit interview with the inspector/auditor will be conducted in order to review observations and general outcomes of the inspection/audit [3].

Possible Findings of the Audit/Inspection

You should be aware of the following routine audit/inspection observations [6]:

- over-delegation by the PI to inappropriately qualified staff
- informed consent process not followed
- informed consent form does not contain the essential elements specified by ICH–GCP
- safety reports not submitted to IRB/IEC
- staff not qualified or trained
- improper storage of records
- lack of SOPs
- inaccurate and/or incomplete records
- clinical trial not conducted in accordance with the protocol

Aspects	What will be reviewed
Clinical research team	• Capability of the clinical research team to conduct the clinical trial • Degree of delegation by the principal investigator • Roles and responsibilities
Protocol	• Trial design, rationale, objectives, treatment plan, and schedule • Investigational product information and dose-modification plans • Study-specific procedures and skill sets • Subject eligibility criteria (inclusion/exclusion) • Registration or randomization procedures • Medical care and ongoing monitoring of trial subjects • Protocol amendments • Multicenter trial procedures • Recruitment strategy and targets • Subject recruitment, enrollment, and tracking • Subject withdrawal criteria and procedures for premature withdrawal • Safety issues • Hazardous waste procedures • Criteria for premature termination or suspension of the trial • Final reporting requirements of the principal investigator
Informed consent process	• Informed consent forms • Documentation of the informed consent process • Subject confidentiality process • Medical care of subjects • Protection of subjects' rights, safety, and wellbeing • Risks subjects are exposed to
Privacy	• Protection of subjects' private or personal health information
IRB/IEC interactions	• Ongoing communication with the IRB/IEC • IRB/IEC approvals • Ethical considerations relating to the trial • IRB/IEC reports

Table 8. Aspects of research conduct and research procedures examined in the audit process. CRF: case report form; FDA: US Food and Drug Administration; ICH-GCP: International Conference on Harmonisation guidelines for Good Clinical Practice; IEC: independent ethics committee; IRB: institutional review board; QA: quality assurance; QC: quality control.

Aspects	What will be reviewed
Communication process	• Subjects • IRB/IEC • Sponsor • Staff • Inspectors • Notes to file • All communication records (eg, fax transmission sheets)
Laboratory procedures	• Adequacy of supplies • Sample collection, processing, and shipping processes • Local or central laboratory certifications • Laboratory reports, follow-up assessments, and medical care
Safety reporting	• Safety information and reporting procedures • Serious adverse event reporting • Unexpected adverse event reporting • Adverse drug reaction reporting • Investigational new drug reports • Sponsor communications and follow-up
Investigational product	• Supply, handling, and storage of the investigational product accountability • Labeling of the investigational product • Compliance with Good Manufacturing Practice • Investigational product/study drug accountability instructions • Dispensing process • Investigational product documentation and records
Data collection	• QA and QC procedures • CRF completion and accuracy • Validation of data from CRF to source documents • CRF collection process • Overall data management process • Overall study data • Site records and documentation • Accuracy and completeness of the study data • Data trail • Electronic data systems • Study files • Data storage and retention

Table 8. *Continued.*

Aspects	What will be reviewed
Records	• Subject recruitment and enrollment logs • Drug accountability/dispensing records • Direct access requirements to source data/documents • Data handling and record keeping • Data retention process • Organization system for all records • Record storage and retention
Essential documents (these are covered in more detail in **Chapter 9**)	• Regulatory binder or regulatory file box • All ICH-GCP essential documents • System used to organize documents
Monitoring	• Monitoring procedures and timing • Monitoring reports • Site visit log • Ongoing communication process with sponsor
Contracts	• Site and sponsor contract obligations and signatures • Letter of agreement • Indemnification agreement • Site's and sponsor's financial obligations • Payment schedule and tracking • Publication policy
Regulatory and compliance	• Audit/inspection plans and procedures • Standard operating procedures • Good Clinical Practice guidelines • QA and QC • Good Manufacturing Practice • Good Laboratory Practice • Regulation review (eg, of applicable FDA regulations)

Table 8. *Continued.*

Conclusion

After much scrutiny of the clinical research industry over the last few years, site visits and audits/inspections are becoming more frequent. The CRC has an important role as a manager, working with the monitor and representatives of contract research organizations in order to monitor the entire clinical trial process.

References

1. International Conference on Harmonisation of Technical Requirements for Registration of Pharmaceuticals for Human Use. ICH Harmonised Tripartite Guideline: Guideline for Good Clinical Practice. E6. Available from: www.ich.org. Accessed November 17, 2004.

2. Paula Jones-Wright, ClinCoach Inc. Clinical Research Coordinator Training: Get Involved in Clinical Research! How to Become a Research Coordinator Course, 2005.

3. Paula Jones-Wright, ClinCoach Inc. Standard Operating Procedures for Clinical Research Sites, 2005.

4. EU Clinical Trials Directive. Available from: www.europa.eu.int/eur-lex/en/search/search_lif.html. Accessed February 10, 2005.

5. Health Canada, Therapeutic Products Directorate. Food and Drug Regulations for Clinical Trials. Division 5. Canada Gazette Part II, 2001;135(13).

6. Health Canada, Health Products and Food Branch Inspectorate. Summary Report of the Inspections of Clinical Trials Conducted under Voluntary Phase, 2003. Available from: www.hc-sc.gc.ca/hpfb-dgpsa/inspectorate/gcp_inspection_sum_rep_e.pdf. Accessed 16 February, 2005.

Chapter 11

Communication

Susan Davie

Introduction

When we communicate we impart or exchange knowledge, thoughts, feelings, or ideas. We do this using speech, writing, expressions, or gestures. There are many ways to get a message across: we can communicate in a face-to-face encounter, use a telephone or fax machine, write an e-mail or letter, or use media such as newspapers, radio, television, and the Internet. As a clinical research coordinator (CRC), you might need to employ all of these methods of communication to successfully organize and bring together every aspect of clinical research conduct into one harmonious operation.

It is important to properly consider the issue of effective communication when planning a clinical research study, since there are so many levels on which the clear and concise exchange of ideas can have a positive impact on the daily management of a study. Indeed, it is far too easy for a lack of clear communication to lead to problems that can cause the whole study to suffer. For example:

- Misunderstandings between research team members can lead to inefficiencies in study conduct that could affect the integrity of the data and the safety of participants.
- Likewise, a failure to communicate clearly during the informed consent process can lead to participants withdrawing their consent and dropping out of the study.
- Even more seriously, the miscommunication of adverse events (AEs) could potentially endanger the safety of other participants.

Therefore, it is extremely important to take the issue of communication seriously.

Communicating with the Research Team

As the CRC, you are the pivotal member of the research team when it comes to the day-to-day running of clinical trials [1]. Therefore, the success or failure of a study will depend on your skills and enthusiasm. Clinical trials are a team effort and, usually, it will be you who keeps the team informed about the study's progress.

Your responsibilities will vary from site to site and can involve a number of jobs. At some sites you may contribute to protocol writing and case report form (CRF) design. The more common tasks you will be expected to undertake involve preparation of the ethics submission, patient recruitment and retention, and the day-to-day running of all research activities [2]. You might also be involved in negotiations with pharmaceutical companies – you could be expected to contribute to discussions about timelines and patient recruitment strategies, and could also help with budget negotiation (although budget negotiation should be the responsibility of other members of the team, you may have an important contribution to make in this area). Such responsibilities will present you with the challenge of communicating in an efficient manner with a multidisciplinary team of people.

Each member of the research team has a different level of responsibility within the trial and to ensure the safety and wellbeing of the research participants, the quality of the data, and the timely completion of the project, you must communicate effectively with them all.

The Principal Investigator

It is vital for you to have open and effective lines of communication with the principal investigator (PI). The PI is often very busy and it is likely that he/she will rely heavily on you for the smooth running of the study. However, you must be able to regularly discuss the project with the PI and have any questions answered satisfactorily.

To achieve this, it is important to arrange regular, frequent meetings with the PI to discuss study-related issues. These meetings do not need to take up a lot of time – a recommendation is 10–15 minutes per day for the duration of the study – and you should bring a list of items that need to be addressed, as well as any documents that need the PI's signature. This will help to save both your time and that of the PI, and will focus the PI's attention on the most important current issues in the study.

You also need to be aware that the PI has a responsibility to impart factual, reasonable, and appropriate information to participants to keep them informed [3]. It is likely that you will play a vital role in this interaction. You will often reinforce and clarify information that the PI has given to study participants, as well as answer any questions that arise.

Study participants may feel more at ease speaking to you and they may direct more questions to you than to the PI. It is important that you and the PI have discussed all aspects of the study and provide consistent information to the study participants. Frequent meetings with the PI will facilitate this.

The Study Monitor

If the clinical trial is sponsored by a company, you will communicate with the company via a designated study monitor (also known as a clinical research associate), who will act as the primary contact person for the sponsor or contract research organization.

You will spend time liaising with the designated monitor to ensure that all regulatory aspects of the trial are in order. This usually involves regular visits to the study site by the monitor. These visits enable him/her to monitor all study-related documentation; this includes comparing study data in case report forms with information in source documents, ensuring that participants are eligible to take part in the study, and ensuring that all ethical aspects of the study are adhered to. The role of the monitor is discussed in more detail in **Chapter 10**.

Because it is essential for CRCs to work closely with monitors, and since the interaction between the two can be time consuming, tensions can arise when there are deadlines to meet. However, it is important to remember that the monitor is also trying to achieve the accurate and timely completion of the study, and is also part of the research team.

The smooth running of the study will be best achieved if both you and the monitor are able to focus clearly on your roles [4]. You should view the monitor as a resource person for the study, as he/she will have a very good working knowledge of the protocol. Monitoring visits should be helpful, particularly early in the study, to reduce any issues with protocol violations or deviations [5].

The best kind of relationship to have with a monitor is one that is open and communicative, and that encourages collaboration – this will make for a positive and professional partnership for the duration of the study. The monitor will make regular visits to the site to monitor the study, and these visits should be at times when information can be exchanged by both you and the monitor. You will both gain the most benefit from monitoring visits if you are prepared by ensuring that everything the monitor will need for the visit is available, eg, completed CRFs, source documents, and the regulatory binder. You should spend some time prior to each visit getting everything up-to-date and ready.

It is critical for the monitor to make a number of visits early on, once the study has been activated and the first one or two participants have been enrolled. This early study monitoring and communication is important because it will reduce the number of mistakes repeated in subsequent data collected during the study [5]. Remember that the monitor will have a good knowledge of the protocol and should be able to answer any questions, either immediately or after having sourced the information. The number and frequency of monitoring visits will, in part, be determined by the rate of enrollment at a particular site.

It is also very important for you to maintain regular communication with the monitor to keep him/her informed of any issues that arise in the day-to-day running of the study. This is particularly important if there are any problems that impact the conduct of the trial either at the site or more broadly, eg, the PI has to change, or a mistake is detected in the CRF. Remember, the monitor needs to be kept informed of such issues in order to provide any assistance that you might need to successfully complete the trial.

Ethics Committees

Institutional review boards (IRBs)/independent ethics committees (IECs) have a fundamental role in the oversight of clinical trials. Often, you will shoulder the workload associated with ethics applications and the ongoing communication associated with the smooth running of the study. It is vital for you to have an open line of communication with the IRB/IEC.

It s recommended that you should prospectively set up routine meetings with the IRB/IEC's administrative office to regularly discuss issues that might arise. IRB/IEC offices that are well staffed will be open to this type of short, routine meeting, which is designed to improve communication and increase efficiency.

When does the communication take place?	What is communicated?
Submission of study to IRB/IEC	Initial IRB/IEC application
	Response to any questions
	Approval or denial of permission to conduct study
Ongoing communications from the study team	Protocol amendments
	Changes to investigators
	Adverse events
	Annual study report
End of study	Final study report

Table 1. A summary of the most common times at which you will communicate with the institutional review board (IRB)/independent ethics committee (IEC).

When making contact with an IRB/IEC to ensure that any changes to submissions or clarification of other issues are being dealt with appropriately, it is often quicker and more useful to speak to the administrative office than to anyone on the IRB/IEC's committee. Having said that, the administrative office is usually extremely busy, resulting in some issues not always being communicated clearly.

All study-specific communication should be in writing and a copy filed in the regulatory binder. By establishing and maintaining a good, open working relationship with the IRB/IEC's administrative office, you will become more efficient and have more time to concentrate on other duties, and will also save the IRB/IEC time. Of course, the administrative office staff should feel the same way about approaching you when there are any issues: open and friendly lines of communication can save a lot of time if questions can be clarified prospectively. The most common times at which you will need to communicate with the IRB/IEC are summarized in **Table 1**.

Adverse Events

It is vital that the IRB/IEC is made aware of AEs and, particularly, serious adverse events (SAEs) in a timely manner. Each institution and IRB/IEC will have their own guidelines for AE reporting. Usually there is a *pro forma* that will be completed by the study team to provide the IRB/IEC with the information it requires, although some IRB/IECs may only require the AE pages of the CRF. This paperwork is essential to ensure that the IRB/IEC is appropriately informed. However, significant

SAEs may initially be reported to the IRB/IEC verbally by a member of the study team, then followed up with the written documentation. This can be important if the required paperwork will take some time to complete: the IRB/IEC will appreciate knowing that there has been a problem with a study participant.

If the PI and study team think that there may be significant problems with the continuation of the study then they should inform the IRB/IEC immediately. Likewise, if the IRB/IEC feels that the study should be suspended or halted then they should immediately contact the study team. You should be aware of the regulatory guidelines relating to AE reporting. It is particularly important to ensure that all AEs are reported not only to the IRB/IEC, but also to the regulatory authority and sponsor (as appropriate).

Primary-care Physicians

Maintaining open lines of communication with participants' primary-care physicians can have a positive impact on study recruitment. Primary-care physicians need to be reassured that referring patients to studies will not result in them losing these patients to other physicians – otherwise, they may be reluctant to refer them to research studies.

As soon as a participant consents to taking part in the study, his/her primary-care physician should be informed; as the CRC, you will often need to ensure that this is done. Primary-care physicians can be an asset during the course of a study. This can be especially evident when the study protocol dictates restrictions on treatments, eg, on medicines that can be co-prescribed with the study drug. You should also ensure that when a participant leaves a research study, his/her primary-care physician is informed and any relevant details are communicated, eg, a change of regular medication.

Other Departments

Since you will often be given the task of organizing the various members of the study team, you should make it a priority to form good relationships with all groups and departments with whom the study team will interact during the duration of a research study. You may frequently be called on to act as a resource person to ensure that all study procedures are carried out in accordance with the protocol, eg, the protocol might dictate that certain procedures are performed in a prescribed way that is slightly different to normal practice.

Resource Departments

Clinical drug trials will usually involve coordination with the pharmacy at the research site. It is a good idea to give the pharmacy prior notice of participants' study visits, particularly if the study requires a complicated dispensing procedure. This will not only help the pharmacy to prepare properly, but will also be beneficial for the participants as they will not have to wait for an extended time to collect their study medicines. Another example is when radiological procedures are necessary: some prior warning for the staff in the radiology department will help to ensure that your trial participants are dealt with quickly and experience minimal waiting times.

Minimizing waiting times for all procedures is important as participants in trials are *volunteers*. After all, study procedures can be time intensive enough, so if participants have to spend more time than is necessary waiting for various tests then they might be reluctant to continue taking part in the study. A smooth-running experience – which is likely to contribute to improved participant retention – can be achieved by forward planning and by communicating with the various areas that you will be utilizing.

Grants Office

In larger centers you might need to liaise with a grants office; this is particularly important for studies that are not industry sponsored. It is vital to communicate regularly with this office to keep abreast of current funding opportunities. The office staff will be aware of the funding sources available for research projects, whether from government or philanthropic agencies. The grants office may have a regular newsletter, often sent via e-mail, and it is important to ensure that you are on the mailing list.

Research Administration Office

Large institutions may have a research administration office. The role of this office can be quite broad, eg, they may offer help with getting project proposals together, applying for funding, and administering the ethics process. You should have a close relationship with the staff from this office, as you may need help at various stages of the study. It is also important to be informed of any changes in the way that research projects are managed at the center, eg, the forms that need to be submitted to the research office may be updated. If you are in regular contact with the research administration office, the office will ensure that any updates or changes are communicated in a timely manner.

Public Relations

In larger centers, another department that can provide an important service is that of public relations (PR). You should ensure that the PR department is involved in any publicity about the research projects you are working on. Publicity can be worthwhile for various reasons:

- You may need to find volunteers to take part in a project, or to let the community know about exciting results.
- On a broader scale, you may receive some positive coverage for the institution carrying out the research.

Open and friendly communication with the PR department can provide opportunities for you to get a message to the community, ie, if PR personnel know who you are and what projects you are working on then they may contact you when they have opportunities for publicity. The PR staff are also a great resource to help with press releases and other advertising strategies; publicity can help to raise the profile of the institution and make it easier to recruit for your particular study

Coordinating Center/Project Coordinator

If the research project is a multicenter study then you will need to communicate with the coordinating center or the overall project coordinator. It might be worthwhile to establish a regular weekly time to make contact with the person who is overseeing the study, whether by phone or regular e-mail update

Intra-departmental Communication

Within the department or research group undertaking the project, regular research meetings are also vital and you could be the pivotal person who ensures that everyone is kept up-to-date about the status of the study. These meetings need to be held regularly, either weekly or every 2 weeks, and an exchange of information should take place between the various people within the research group.

Communicating with Research Participants

Perhaps the most important communication that needs to take place is between the research team and the study participants [3]. This relationship is fostered by an appropriate exchange of study-related information. Participants might initially learn about the study from a variety of sources, eg, flyers in their primary-care physician's office, posters, advertising in the media, Web-based advertising or information, or through a discussion with their primary-care physician.

Once you have made contact with the potential study participant, it is absolutely vital that an honest, open relationship is fostered – this relationship has an enormous influence on the participant's continued contribution to the study.

The first consultation with a potential participant can be crucial in setting the tone for all future communication and study interactions involving him/her [6], so it should be as friendly, informative, and unhurried as possible. This is not always easy in a busy clinic or in a hospital setting, but because this meeting will often decide the outcome of whether a new participant decides to enroll in a study, it is worth doing everything you can to initiate a positive and trusting relationship.

This can be achieved by ensuring that:

- study visits take place in a quiet office
- participants have the opportunity to ask questions
- adequate answers are provided

Providing a reasonable amount of time to ensure that participants have a sound understanding of the requirements of the study will ensure their continued involvment. This will also help to create a trusting relationship as participants will have a good understanding of how the study is planned to unfold.

Informed Consent

You will often have primary responsibility for conducting the process of obtaining informed consent from study participants, and this is the most important occasion on which to clearly communicate information. Even when the consent process is carried out by another team member, you will often be called on by participants to discuss consent-related issues: you might be asked to clarify issues to the participant with regard to informed consent. This often occurs when participants do not fully understand what is expected of them at each visit. You should not underestimate the importance of clear explanation and repetition of explanations given by the PI and other trial staff.

Your role during the informed consent process can develop into one of participant advocacy, and so open and clear communication, as well as developing a trusting relationship with the study participant, are vital for this to take place appropriately.

You must be able to clearly explain all aspects of the trial and what is expected of the participant. This can involve a large amount of – sometimes very technical – information. It is especially important to be able to describe all aspects of the trial in understandable language, without using too many technical words or medical jargon, and to make sure that any unfamiliar words or phrases are fully explained to the participant. Individual IRBs/IECs may have guidelines detailing the level of language that is acceptable, and you should familiarize yourself with these.

Good aids to communication include the following:

- When talking with participants, it helps to have a quiet room where there will be no interruptions.
- There should be a comprehensive, written participant information statement and informed consent document detailing all aspects of the study.
- The potential participant should be given adequate time to read the documents and to ask any questions that he/she or his/her family members might have.

Other approaches and aids can also be used to help explain procedures or to describe how the study will affect those taking part – eg, anatomical models, or videos of the study procedures or the informed consent process might be of use. Both you and the participant can find these to be a valuable aid to communication and understanding.

Another useful way of conveying study-related information to participants is to give them an outline of what will happen at each visit and an estimate of the amount of time each visit will take. Although the informed consent document should contain this, it is helpful to create an additional quick guide for easy reference. This is particularly helpful if there are special requirements for certain visits, such as the need to fast for blood tests.

Once a participant has signed the informed consent document, you should ensure that you or some other appropriate person (such as the PI) is available to answer questions and to deal with problems at any time during the study period.

You should make certain that all participants know how to get in touch if they need to, and are made to feel that they can do so at any time. A wallet-sized card displaying the study title and contact details for study staff will be useful for participants and is also helpful for other healthcare workers in the case of an emergency.

Withdrawal of Consent

Participants also need to be aware that they can terminate their consent to take part in the study at any time. If a participant is not happy to continue, for any reason, it is important that they are comfortable with letting the PI know that they wish to withdraw their consent. This can be helpful for both parties, as just leaving a trial may be a problem for the participant, particularly if they should wean off the study medication and not cease it suddenly. It can also be beneficial to the study team, as there may be some end of study or study termination procedures to complete at the final visit.

Cultural Differences and Special Populations

When communicating with participants, you need to take into consideration any cultural differences between you and the participants, be they language, religious, or other lifestyle issues. It is vital that an approved interpreter is employed if the potential participant does not speak the same language as members of the research team, and you should ensure that you know how to make effective use of the interpreter.

Religious and Cultural Differences

Religious and other lifestyle choices need to be handled with sensitivity, and open lines of communication are very important to ensure that all issues are dealt with appropriately. For example, there can be times when the participant will not be available, or when it may not be appropriate for a participant to be unescorted by a family member. Your role will be made easier if cultural concerns are respected and dealt with, with a minimum of disruption to both you and the participant.

Specific issues will vary widely from country to country, and there may even be regional differences within countries. Most differences will involve religious beliefs and, even within the major religions, beliefs and traditions can vary depending on where in the world people live.

It is important for you to have a good knowledge of the cultural and ethnic groups within your community. If you are unsure of what is acceptable, you should make this clear to the potential participant by asking a simple question about whether he/she has any restrictions that might affect his/her participation in the study. If you are unsure about the traditions of a particular group then a quick search on the Internet might give you some information – this can also act as a place to start a dialogue about cultural restrictions.

Vulnerable Populations

Special care also needs to be taken with research involving vulnerable populations. This includes [7]:

- emergency care research
- intensive care research
- neonatal intensive care research
- pediatric research (see below)
- terminal care research
- research involving people with impaired capacity for communication
- research involving unconscious people
- research involving people with an intellectual or mental impairment

When dealing with these groups during research, it is very important that you develop appropriate lines of communication with the study participants. This will need to be assessed on a case-by-case basis, but if you are not experienced in dealing with a specific participant population then you should seek guidance from colleagues who are experienced with these groups.

Any form of communication may be impossible with some groups, eg, neonates or unconscious participants. The level of special care taken might need to be enhanced further if a participant's family is involved, or in situations involving possible surrogate consent.

Pediatric Populations

The pediatric population will provide you with specialized challenges. When working with children, the primary concern is to determine their capacity for understanding, since this varies across age groups and between individuals [8]. This is an extra challenge as the IRB/IEC might require parental consent and/or participant assent. There are no hard and fast rules when dealing with children, and each child needs to be assessed individually: some 8-year-olds will understand more than some 15-year-olds. You should endeavor to build a rapport with the child to decide what level of information to communicate to them.

It is important that all aspects of the study are explained to the child and it is worthwhile for you to prepare for any discussion by planning how to explain the study requirements in a simple way. You should also be aware that children are perceptive and will pick up signals if you are not being honest or not disclosing enough information.

The opportunity to ask questions is important and allowing time for this to happen is vital. It may be appropriate to take some time out to play a game or to do some craft work with the child; this will help to create a non-threatening environment and give the child a chance to set their own agenda with any discussion that they might like to have. It can be helpful to leave the office or examination room and spend time in an area that is dedicated to play. It may also be useful to give adolescents some space away from their parents to have a discussion about the study – this is especially important if you are unsure whether the adolescent really wants to take part.

Issues of pediatric informed consent and assent are discussed further in **Chapter 6**.

International Communications

CRCs in all of the International Conference on Harmonisation regions must be effective communicators in order to achieve the best outcomes for the projects they are working on. However, one of the major problems encountered when CRCs are involved in international research projects is time differences between the different regions of the globe. This can be easily overcome if the regions have an overlap in business hours, but it becomes more difficult if the time zones do not overlap at all (eg, when everyone is at work in Australia it is nighttime in the USA).

This is problematic if there is an SAE that might have an impact on the ongoing safety of study participants as it is vital for the information to be disseminated to the sponsor and onto the participating investigator sites as quickly as possible. With time-zone differences, there can be a delay in this important information reaching everyone who should be informed. Of course, this information can be distributed as quickly as possible via e-mail.

Conclusion

Overall, your communication skills are vital to the harmonious running of clinical research. In all aspects of trial coordination, your skill as an open and effective communicator will assist with the timely completion of clinical studies, thus benefiting all those involved in the process. You should also act as a study team coordinator, incorporating all of the various study contributors into the overall team. In many ways, you have to be all things to all people. Your tasks will include:

- helping the PI focus on the study
- keeping the monitor informed about the ongoing management of the study
- dealing with the IRB/IEC
- liaising with other departments
- (most importantly) providing effective communication about the study to the study participants

To achieve this you must employ a variety of skills: verbal, written, and organizational – you must be diplomatic, and you should set goals to achieve the best outcomes for all those involved in the research studies that you are working on.

References

1. Fedor C, Cola P. Preliminary results of the Clinical Researcher coordinators' survey. Clinical Researcher 2003;3(4):18-22.

2. Neuer A. The rising tide of CRC workload and turnover. CenterWatch 2002;(8):1-7.

3. Sorensen JB, Rossel P, Holm S. Patient-physician communication concerning participation in cancer chemotherapy trials. Br J Cancer 2004;90:328-32.

4. Cola P. The Coordinators' Forum. A need to refine suitable roles for CRC's and CRA's. Clinical Researcher 2004;4(6):4 (unpublished).

5. Holland L. The Coordinators' Forum. Communication is key to the CRC-CRA team. Clinical Researcher 2004;4(6):3 (unpublished).

6. Shannon C. Better communication is key to recruiting patients to trials. BMJ 2003;327:1368.

7. National Health and Medical Research Council. National Statement on Ethical Conduct in Research Involving Humans. Commonwealth of Australia 2001. Available from: www.nhmrc.gov.au/publications/titles.htm. Accessed November 22, 2004.

8. Fedor C, Houston J. The Coordinators' Forum Part 7: Children as research participants - historical, ethical and practical perspectives. Clinical Researcher 2002;2(10):26-8.

Chapter 12

Learning: a Continuous Journey

Andrea G Procaccino

Introduction

As a clinical research coordinator (CRC), you are a critical component of responsible research conduct and the success of the clinical research you are involved in revolves around you. Why is this? The investigator will often rely on you to carry out most of the major activities involved in conducting a trial, and so the education, training, and continuous learning opportunities you receive become critical. The better educated and trained you are, the higher the quality of the trial will be.

If a major part of the study burden is to be placed on the CRC's shoulders, it is necessary for the clinical research industry to ensure that you are given the proper tools to be successful. Education and training are the first tools that CRCs should be given for their clinical research toolbox.

The training requirements of each CRC will differ, as they will largely depend on the site and trial, in addition to your own personal requirements. Currently, there is no mandatory certification for CRCs, and available learning opportunities can vary considerably according to the site and the clinical trial [1–3]. Most training will occur 'on the job', and you will often have to identify your own training needs and seek out training opportunities [4,5].

It is important to note that learning is a continuous process and not a one-time event. The clinical research industry never stands still [5]. New opportunities for promotion and progression can appear, which might require you to learn new skills, although these will depend on your site. Once experienced as a CRC, it is

Educational background of coordinators with a graduate qualification	Percentage of respondents
Medicine	21.6
Nursing	16.2
Pharmacy	13.5
Biology	13.5
Other	19.0
Total coordinators with a university degree	83.8

Table 1. Educational backgrounds of respondents to a survey of 41 clinical research coordinators involved in oncology clinical trials in Spain. Copyright © 2004 Rico-Villademoros et al; licensee BioMed Central Ltd [3].

likely that you will also be expected to provide training to other members of the clinical research team, and so it is useful to have an understanding of the key principles of effective adult education.

In this chapter, the various types of training and continuous learning that are available to you will be explored, as will the role that you might play in training others.

Entering the Fray

The previous experience and backgrounds of new CRCs are diverse, although they often have a background in healthcare and some level of basic medical knowledge and/or therapeutic expertise (see **Table 1**) [2–4,6–8]. However, it is unlikely that new CRCs will have had previous training and/or experience in trial coordination as, when hiring new CRCs, employers often consider previous experience to be less important than more general project management skills [1].

Responsibilities and Skills

The clinical investigator will share with you the responsibility for making sure that the appropriate regulations are followed, the mandates of the protocol are adhered to, and the trial is conducted accurately and is ethically sound. Put simply, you can make or break a clinical study.

You will contribute to all of the critical elements of research conduct, including subject recruitment and retention, direct subject care, and study logistics, as well as performing roles as diverse as managing the relationship with the sponsor and acting as primary study contact, research site administrator, motivator, facilitator, mediator, coach, and confidante, to name just a few possibilities (a more comprehensive discussion of the CRC's role can be found in **Chapter 1**). The site you work at, and the team you work with, will dictate the exact tasks that you will need to carry out and, consequently, the particular skills you must develop.

Requirements for Training

Given the critical role that the CRC plays in ensuring the responsible conduct of research, it is no coincidence that the International Conference on Harmonisation guidelines for Good Clinical Practice (ICH–GCP) state that personnel involved in the conduct of clinical trials must be qualified to perform their respective tasks by education, training, and experience [9]. Although ICH–GCP does not specify the form that such education, training, and experience should take, this will be evaluated during monitoring visits and ICH–GCP inspections by reviewing the research team's CVs/résumés in the light of their trial responsibilities [8].

Identifying Training Needs

Despite the importance of the CRC's responsibilities, many CRCs receive little or no standardized instruction or training before being introduced into their clinical research role [1]. Instead, the usual introduction to coordination is to learn 'on the job' [2,4,5]. The training needs of established study team members can be identified by considering the research team's experience in the context of the protocol-specific skills that are required, and by recognizing any previous areas of weakness identified by monitoring [8].

Opportunities for Training

In a perfect world, new CRCs would be initiated through an extensive training and orientation program. This would enable them to learn the fundamentals and practical applications of GCP, followed immediately by extensive protocol-specific training provided by the sponsor company. In reality, however, the first training that a new CRC receives is usually on-the-job training from another CRC.

While on-the-job training is usually available at any site, some sites might also offer other, longer-term learning opportunities: some sites will offer on-site workshops, or the chance to attend off-site seminars, while others might offer no formal training at all [1,2]. Even if your site offers no opportunities for training, there may be other opportunities that you can pursue independently, eg, by making use of e-learning resources, or by becoming certified. Some commonly encountered training methods are discussed below.

On-the-Job Training

The format of on-the-job training will vary from site to site, because at different sites different people are responsible for teaching new CRCs. Staff members with responsibility for training new CRCs can include:

- the investigator, as he/she is ultimately responsible for the training of study site staff [9]
- a senior CRC, who might act as a mentor
- a specialist trainer, although this is more likely if the site runs a formal training program

Often, on-the-job training is provided by a CRC, who might be too busy to devote the amount of training time that is truly needed. In order for on-the-job training to be effective, dedicated and skilled trainers should be paired-up with new CRCs – these trainers should act as coaches and mentors as well as being personal tutors. Mentoring is discussed in further detail in **Chapter 4**.

On-the-job training is important to the overall education process, but it should not be the sole element. It should be balanced with other forms of learning; people given the responsibility to deliver on-the-job training are often experts in their fields, but this does not mean that they can effectively communicate this knowledge to another person.

Classroom Instruction

Classroom instruction is an optimal situation because it provides a chance for people to interact with their peers, who will be experiencing similar situations or challenges, and it is also a good networking opportunity. The classroom instructor should be skilled at evaluating learners' understanding of the material and ensuring that there is indeed a transfer of knowledge.

Classroom training also provides opportunities for the hands-on application of concepts through audience participation, discussions, asking questions, and problem-solving [10], which will help learners to retain the new knowledge. There are many training organizations supporting the pharmaceutical and medical device

Name	Country	Website
Traditional learning		
American Academy of Pharmaceutical Physicians	USA	www.aapp.org
Association for Clinical Data Management	UK	www.acdm.org.uk
Association of Clinical Research Professionals	International	www.acrpnet.org
British Association of Research Quality Assurance	UK	www.barqa.com
ClinCoach, Inc.	Canada	www.clincoach.com
Drug Information Association	International	www.diahome.org
Public Responsibility in Research and Medicine	USA	www.primr.org
Society of Clinical Research Associates	USA	www.socra.org
US Department of Health and Human Services Office of Research Integrity	USA	www.ori.hhs.gov/conferences
E-learning		
ClinPhone Group Ltd		www.clinphone.com
Hurley Write, Inc.		www.hurleywrite.com
Pharmaforsite		www.pharmaforsite.com
The RAN Institute		www.raninstitute.com

Table 2. Examples of organizations, professional associations, and companies that provide clinical research training, workshops, and seminars.

industries, as well as professional associations that provide classroom seminars and workshops on topics that directly affect CRCs (see **Table 2**).

Useful learning topics for the classroom that are of relevance to CRCs might include (to name but a few):

- an introduction to GCP
- topics for new CRCs
- topics for intermediate CRCs
- topics for advanced CRCs
- subject recruitment and retention
- how to write standard operating procedures

The ACRP exam for recognition as a Certified CRC is comprised of 125 multiple-choice questions covering study activities, prestudy activities, study management, and study termination, and it is held at locations throughout the world. In order to take the exam, candidates must have a minimum of 2 years' experience of working as a CRC. The ACRP requires Certified CRCs to recertify every 2 years. This process involves the completion of 24 continuing education contact hours, of which 50% must be in clinical research-oriented training courses, home study programs, or symposia/conferences, while the remainder can be contributed from other approved sources within the healthcare field.

Table 3. Association of Clinical Research Professionals (ACRP) certification [11]. CRC: clinical research coordinator.

E-learning

We are all passengers on the current technological information highway. As a result, there are opportunities for training and learning to take place whenever and wherever it is needed. There are many vendors of e-learning materials, which can take the form of computer-based training modules, simulation modules, and Web-based learning sites (see **Table 2**). The advantage that e-learning offers is that the training is available 24 hours a day, 7 days a week, and can be accessed conveniently – training can be taken in a step-by-step fashion whenever a window of time presents itself.

Certification

Certification is one trend that continues to shape the future training landscape for CRCs. A number of certification programs have emerged for clinical research associates (monitors), CRCs, and, more recently, clinical investigators. The first certification program for CRCs was begun in 1990 by the Association for Clinical Research Professionals (ACRP) in the USA (see **Table 3**).

To date, ACRP has certified over 9,500 clinical research coordinators and now offers certification directed at the international clinical research community at locations worldwide [11]. The Society of Clinical Research Associates also offers certification for all levels of clinical research professionals (see **Table 4**) [12], while the American Academy of Pharmaceutical Physicians and the Drug Information Association offer certification directed primarily at investigators. These programs formally recognize a CRC's professional experience in addition to their performance in a certification exam.

Certification has become very important because it offers a documented assurance of knowledge of GCP, and the regulations and guidelines that protect human research subjects. In order to receive National Institutes of Health (NIH) funding

The SoCRA standard of Certified Clinical Research Professional (CCRP) is open to any professional within the clinical research arena who meets certain standards. As with the Association of Clinical Research Professionals (ACRP) certification, SoCRA requires professionals to have 2 years' experience of clinical trials in order to qualify. The written examination covers five major subject areas:

- conduct of clinical trials
- institutional review boards and regulations
- ethical issues
- ability to follow directions
- abstracting information from medical records

Unlike the ACRP exam, the SoCRA exam must be renewed after 3 years, by means of 45 hours of continuing education credit and a recertification quiz. SoCRA currently have 3,667 certified CCRP members (Erich Lukas, SoCRA, personal communication, January 2005).

Table 4. Society of Clinical Research Associates (SoCRA) certification [12].

for clinical research in the USA, key personnel involved with a trial must have received training in human subjects protections (see **Chapter 3**), and documentation must be submitted to the funding body to demonstrate this. Most institutions now provide their staff with educational courses that fulfill this requirement; in addition, the NIH provides an online educational resource "NIH Human Participant Protections Education for Research Teams" to intramural investigators and research professionals [13].

The training and certification of clinical research professionals might ultimately be required by industry sponsors during site selection as it already is for NIH-funded research in the USA. Indeed it is the logical next step, as human subjects protection programs begin to become accredited throughout the USA, and an increasing number of CRCs and other research professionals attain accreditation. Some sponsor companies provide financial support for CRCs to obtain certification, while others expect CRCs to be proactive and to pursue this certification on their own to increase their marketability.

Maintaining the Momentum

The world of clinical research is forever changing. This is natural: the industry must continue to evolve to keep progressing towards a more stable and stringent set of ethical principles and a state of higher quality to meet the demand for the continuous improvement of global healthcare. Training, education, and learning are

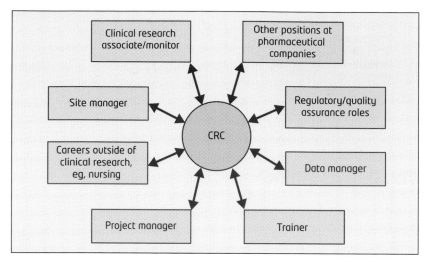

Figure 1. Careers related to clinical research coordinator (CRC) [11,14].

the tools we must use to develop and adapt ourselves, so that we remain valuable to the current international environment and clinical research infrastructure.

We often think of training as a static, one-time event – we attend a course, receive a certificate of completion for that session, and are now thought of as 'trained'. But this is a short-sighted and inaccurate point of view. Although opportunities will depend on your site, training is a continuous process, with each newly acquired piece of knowledge serving as a stepping stone to the next level of career development and advancement. Recertification will require continuing education, accentuating the continuum of learning. Indeed, in today's competitive business environment, your job security will be increasingly dependent on your ability to grow and quickly learn new skills. Today, most adults have to relearn their jobs several times in the life of their career, and in this respect the CRC is no different.

As you become more experienced, you may wish to explore other areas and tasks that you have not tackled before, eg, fiscal and legal aspects of contracts, budgets, taking responsibility for the operating budget, new business development, and writing standard operating procedures. Alternatively, you may wish to take on new roles within clinical research, such as becoming a trainer, clinical research associate, or pharmaceutical company employee, or by focusing on more specialized tasks, eg, data management. Some careers related to that of CRC are given in **Figure 1** and some characteristics most valued by employers are listed in **Table 5**.

• Ability to communicate	• Desire to learn
• Ability to link information, eg, anticipate the impact that a change in a patient's medication might have on the expected adverse events	• Good organization skills
	• Medical background
	• Positive attitude
• Attention to detail	• Self motivated
• Desire to continue caring for patients	

Table 5. Some desired characteristics of clinical research coordinators [1].

The CRC as Trainer

Once you have been recognized as a competent and knowledgeable member of the clinical research team at a site, you will often be called on to act as a trainer for new or more junior staff. Typically, there will not be dedicated training staff to assist you with this additional task, but many coordinators creatively and proactively develop their own research networks or forums for sharing information and knowledge. In essence, by doing this they are establishing their own learning culture amongst their peers. Having said this, to better educate and train your peers, you must understand the basic principles of adult learning.

Basic Principles of Adult Learning

It is a well known fact that children and adults learn differently. Malcolm Knowles first introduced this concept – also known as andragogy – in the 1970s [15]. Although it sparked much controversy at the time of its presentation, it has since come to represent the core principles of adult learning and, in turn, enable those who design and deliver training to adults to build more effective programs. This concept relates to the characteristics of the learning event itself, not to the training event's overall goals. The andragogical model of adult learning is based on the following principles [15]:

- The need to know: adults need to know *why* they must learn something before they learn it. In the situation of training and education, the adult learner needs to know how the learning will be conducted, what will be learned, and why it will be valuable.
- The learner's self-concept: adults have a self-concept of being responsible for their own decisions.

- The role of the learner's experiences: adults come into an educational activity with many previous experiences that need to be considered.
- Readiness to learn: adults become ready to learn those things necessary to help cope with real-life situations. This is also closely associated with the 'need to know' principle.
- Orientation to learning: adults are motivated to learn to the extent that they perceive that learning will help them perform tasks or deal with situations encountered in real-life.
- Motivation: to an adult, the most potent motivators are internal pressures such as self-esteem, quality of life, and increased job satisfaction. Adults look for a 'personal payoff' from learning.

Gibbons has also provided a model that is useful in CRC training, which suggests that learners need to be effective in three types of learning [16]:

1. Natural learning: learning that occurs as the individual interacts spontaneously with the environment. For CRCs, this would translate to on-the-job learning.
2. Formal learning: learning in which the content is chosen by others and presented to the learner. Professional seminars on topics such as GCP and certification preparatory courses would fall into this category.
3. Personal learning: self-directed or intentional learning. This requires the learner to take a proactive approach to obtaining the skills and knowledge he/she needs.

Characteristics of an Effective Trainer

Any CRC who is put in the role of trainer needs to have a basic understanding of adult learning principles. You must take these principles into consideration when designing a new CRC orientation program, or a technical training session on a given skill or task, in order to design and deliver a training event that will have the greatest positive impact on the adult learner. It is not effective simply to pull together information into a slide presentation and deliver it at the front of the room: some thought and planning must be done in order to effectively transfer information to the adult learner in such a fashion as to promote increased comprehension and retention of that knowledge as it relates to his/her function as a CRC.

The CRC must also have the self-confidence and presence to be able to:

- train/present to a group of peers
- keep them engaged and interested in learning more
- listen to what the trainees are saying

Another key asset of a successful trainer is the ability to understand and embrace the fact that the best teachers are the ones who never stop learning. Therefore, trainers must stay current with the regulations and guidelines, and continually challenge and expand their own minds in the same way that they encourage the CRCs they teach to open their minds to new techniques and ideas.

Conclusion

As a CRC, you will often be relied on to carry out most of the major activities involved in conducting a trial, and so it is of vital importance for you to be trained in all aspects of trial conduct. Training should be considered as a continual process and not a one-time event, and new opportunities for promotion and progression might appear, which can require you to learn new skills. Once experienced as a CRC, it is likely that you will also be expected to provide training to other members of the clinical research team, and it is important for you to be educated and trained in this area to ensure that you can effectively fulfill such responsibilities.

Any CRC who is put in the role of trainer needs to have a basic understanding of adult learning principles and must also have the self-confidence and presence to be able to be able to train their peers effectively. The best teachers are the ones who never stop learning – trainers should expand their own minds in the same way that they encourage their students.

Learning is a wonderful journey: it starts at birth and does not end until we take our last breath. Embrace learning, embrace the challenges it presents, and make it a part of every day.

References

1. Borfitz D. CRC loss tied to heavy workload. The CenterWatch Monthly 2004:11(7):1-5. Available from: www.centerwatch.com/careers/CW1107_crc.pdf. Accessed January 2, 2005.

2. Fedor C, Cola P. Preliminary results of the Clinical Researcher coordinators' survey. Clinical Researcher 2003;3(4):18-22.

3. Rico-Villademoros F, Hernando T, Sanzl J-L, et al. The role of the clinical research coordinator – data manager – in oncology clinical trials. BMC Medical Research Methodology 2004:4:6. Available from: www.biomedcentral.com/1471-2288/4/6. Accessed January 2, 2005.

4. Mueller MR. From delegation to specialization: nurses and clinical trial coordination. Nurs Inq 2001;8(3):182-90.

5. Fedor C. The Coordinators' Forum. Part 4: The continuum of learning for coordinators. Clinical Researcher 2002:2(4):24.

6. Davis AM, Hull SC, Grady C, et al. The invisible hand in clinical research: the study coordinator's critical role in human subjects protection. J Law Med Ethics 2002;30(3):411-19.

7. Halloran L. ACRP's North American salary analysis. The Monitor 1998;Winter.

8. Jones-Wright P. Going for gold in clinical research through training and education. Part 1: Understanding the requirements for training and education. Clinical Researcher 2002:2(9):18-21.

9. International Conference on Harmonisation of Technical Requirements for Registration of Pharmaceuticals for Human Use. ICH Harmonised Tripartite Guideline: Guideline for Good Clinical Practice. E6. Available from: www.ich.org. Accessed November 17, 2004.

10. Jones-Wright P. Going for gold in clinical research through training and education. Part 2: Ways to educate and train researchers. Clinical Researcher 2003;3(2):24-9.

11. Association of Clinical Research Professionals (ACRP) Web site. Available from: www.acrpnet.org. Accessed January 2, 2005.

12. Society of Clinical Research Associates (SoCRA) Web site. Available from: www.socra.org/certific.htm. Accessed January 2, 2005.

13. National Institutes of Health. Required Education in the Protection of Human Research Participants. June 5, 2000. Available from: grants.nih.gov/grants/guide/notice-files/NOT-OD-00-039.html. Accessed January 2, 2005.

14. Neuer A. The rising tide of CRC workload and turnover. CenterWatch 2002:9(8):1-7. Available from: www.centerwatch.com/careers/CW0908_CRCTurnover.pdf. Accessed January 3, 2005.

15. Knowles MS, Holton EF, Swanson RA. The Adult Learner: The Definitive Classic in Adult Education and Human Resource Development. 5th ed. Houston, TX: Gulf Professional Publishing, 1998.

16. Gibbons M. A working model of the learning how to learn process. In: Smith RM. Learning How to Learn Across the Life Span. San Francisco, CA: Jossey-Bass, 1990.

Chapter 13

Future Trends: the Professionalization of the CRC

Carol A Fedor

Edward F Gabriele

"...as science speeds ahead, it often pushes the edges of society's readiness to cope with consequences. Increasingly, research creates possibilities before the accompanying ethical, social, and legal ramifications have been resolved" [1].

Introduction

This book reminds us that clinical research is conducted throughout the world and, wherever the site at which it is conducted, great importance is placed on respecting and protecting the safety and rights of human research participants. Principles for the conduct of clinical research are set forth in internationally recognized documents, ie, the International Conference on Harmonisation guidelines for Good Clinical Practice [2]. These principles and other standards for clinical research conduct – eg, the more recent guidelines for the responsible conduct of research discussed in **Chapters 3** and **4** – are translated into legal requirements through laws and regulations enforced by national and local authorities.

As commented by the Pharmaceutical Research and Manufacturers of America, "Many different entities and individuals contribute to the safe and appropriate conduct of clinical research, including not only sponsoring companies, but also regulatory agencies; investigative site staff [including clinical research coordinators

(CRCs)] and medical professionals who serve as clinical investigators; hospitals and other institutions where research is conducted; and institutions review boards and ethics committees" [3]. CRCs are often acknowledged for their significant contribution to clinical research and referred to as 'the heart and soul of the study'. A number of CRC surveys have revealed that CRCs' primary motivations in their role are contributing to the development of new therapies to treat disease and improving the quality of life for research participants.

Over time, the role of the CRC has expanded to include a growing number of job functions, ranging from everyday study tasks to recruitment and marketing, managing the study's finances, marketing the research site, managing data, ensuring compliance of the research conduct, and, most importantly, acting as advocate for the research participant. The role of CRC appears to be adapting *as a result of* trends in clinical research, and these trends continue to lead to further responsibilities that require increased knowledge and expertise across additional and diverse competencies.

Leading the Way

While this increased emphasis on regulatory knowledge and project management skills will help to further professionalize the role of the CRC, we must consider whether the future direction of the CRC profession should, in principle, transform the true meaning of human subjects protection by navigating away from a 'culture of compliance' to a 'culture of integrity'. This would mean that, much like the actual research itself, the CRC would be expected to break new ground and provide leadership, and not simply respond to trends.

Providing leadership in the clinical research environment has historically been thought of as the role of the principal investigator (PI). However, recent trends and research indicate that CRCs contribute to study leadership in an equal or perhaps greater quantity compared with the PI. It is hoped that this book will continue to help the role of the CRC to evolve towards a generalizable profession, which all CRCs can relate to and understand as a position of leadership.

Our experience of clinical research has indicated that CRCs and investigators operate in limited environments particular to their own area of expertise and, generally, they do not cross boundaries into other areas of clinical research or areas outside of clinical research. This limits the role of the CRC to a specific approach and does not necessarily open up the CRC's role to one where leadership is resultant. This book provides particular examples to all CRCs of how these boundaries need to be expanded in order to professionalize the role. For example, issues pertaining to assent should be understood, not merely by CRCs specializing in pediatrics, but rather by all CRCs: the principles of participant assent apply to more than just pediatric research.

Additionally, CRCs need to embrace and understand each area of responsible research conduct, including those that have not always been previously viewed as being within the CRC's realm, eg, conflicts of interest and authorship. Understanding conflicts of interest is likely to help the CRC to comprehend his/her role in a more financial manner and, by understanding the intricacies of authorship, the role of the CRC will be placed squarely within academia. Finally, CRCs need to take a different approach towards regulatory information and study documentation, so that these responsibilities become a necessity by second nature instead of being perceived as potentially hindering the progress of research. These roles are akin to standard approaches taken by professionals in business and legal environments.

A Guiding Ethos

The ultimate outcome measure of the professionalization of the CRC's role and the development of CRC leadership in the conduct of clinical research is the progress of medical science and the protection of human research subjects. CRC's have a responsibility to advance medical science within the confines of particular regulations and guidelines, and under the directions and intentions of those who exercise the ethical authority for human subjects protection. Therefore, CRCs have as their guiding 'ethos' the same ethical foundations as those who have authority for discernment. In the USA at the present time, this ethos is predominantly composed of the hallmarks of human subject protections found in the "Belmont Report" [4].

Arising from a historically interesting set of origins and 5 years of intense work, the "Belmont Report" was issued in 1979 by the National Commission for the Protection of Human Subjects of Biomedical and Behavioral Research. The report identified three hallmarks that today constitute the foundational 'ethos principles' for the protection of human research participants:

- respect for persons and their autonomy
- beneficence
- justice

These hallmarks, or foundational principles, clearly give important shape to the task of clinical research leadership, namely:

- to protect the right of individuals to practice self-determination, and the protection of that right for individuals with diminished autonomy
- to ensure that research is conducted such that human benefit is maximized and risks are minimized
- to guarantee that the risks and benefits of research are not enjoined on or given to one segment of the population unfairly or without proper scientific and humane proportionality

However, these hallmarks are not just another set of abstract principles. They are more akin to what might be constituted by classical philosophy as 'virtues'. In this regard, respect for persons, beneficence, and justice challenge the future role of the CRC and other clinical research leaders to evolve beyond that of professionalism, and to grow based on personal commitment and integrity. These leaders are faced with increasing pressure to advance clinical research, yet must maintain an impeccable level of integrity through the protection of human participant volunteers, in order to sustain the necessary level of trust for such progress.

The Impact of Business

Clinical research in the USA, the EU, and Japan has, for wide and diverse reasons, adopted the industrial model as a means of understanding and shaping what have come to be called best business practices. There is nothing inherently wrong with utilizing the business matrix to seek ways to improve healthcare and the delivery of healthcare research. However, as with all other aspects of human activity, this choice comes at a price.

The price that may have been paid over the last decades is that of a possible distracting or blurring of the fundamental life choice or 'vocation' of the CRC or healthcare professional. Utility in function and the quantification of success through the use of metrics need to be tempered and balanced by continually returning to the roots of clinical research: qualitative human and humane care.

In a utilitarian business environment, the provision of such care cannot necessarily be assumed. The principles of such care are not automatically possessed by new entrants to the healthcare and clinical research workforce, because the fundamental basis of modern society makes it difficult for people to inherently practice these methods without being seen as a roadblock to progress. If it were easier to practice such methods then some of the difficulties that endure despite the increase in regulation might not be in evidence.

Research trends over the last two decades clearly show that investigator-initiated and federally funded research no longer holds the level of prestige in academic circles that it once did. During this time, the advent of enormous amounts of private research funding has clearly increased the focus on industry-sponsored research. Within the pharmaceutical industry, the most important measure of innovation is the extent to which new drugs are developed and marketed. Non-industry-sponsored studies have their own pressures: these relate to the advancement of medical science through levels of federal grant funding, and academic prestige and tenure.

The clinical research industry is confronted by many issues, including a requirement for an increased number of trials, an increased number of participants, the cost of getting an approved drug to market, and the cost of delays in getting a drug to market. On average, it takes 10–15 years and costs more than US$800 million to do the research and testing necessary to bring a new therapy to patients [5].

These business pressures are likely to continue and may result in a more industrial approach to the conduct of clinical research (ie, the continued proliferation of medical science driven by private money, versus a more independent, academic approach; a delicate balance of these two approaches needs to be maintained for the appropriate advancement of medical science).

The impact of this approach is evident in the area of recruitment: As observed by the US Department of Health and Human Services, "...in recent years, the clinical research environment has become more commercialized and competitive... In this changing environment, with significant increases in the number and complexity of clinical trials, the quest to find human subjects has intensified" [6]. The pressures of recruitment fall on the shoulders of the PIs, CRCs, and research sites, who are faced with meeting the sponsor's enrollment deadlines with fewer eligible subjects. This often leads to less time for an individual to complete his/her responsibilities, and increases the potential for error or poor judgment.

Moving Forwards

The recent emphasis on requirements for the certification and education of clinical research professionals has necessitated more protected time for training, yet findings of research misconduct have continued to increase in frequency [7]. This implies that the training of individuals who are already in the field is inadequate on its own. Professional training in clinical research needs to begin sooner, ie, during training for healthcare-related professions. Universities, and other training institutions for allied health professions, need to recognize and plan curricula in the area of clinical research, so that an individual has the fundamentals in place prior to being in the position of conducting clinical research. Also, clinical research job positions and continuing education opportunities need to become standardized at institutions and not be based solely on financial decisions relating to funding levels for research.

However, there may be something far deeper emerging within the culture of research that will affect and expand, in quantum leap fashion, the mission of CRCs and similar healthcare or research professionals. Over more than the past decade, a need has emerged within the research community to reflect on why there continues to be evidence of problems in clinical research, despite the proliferation of regulatory requirements.

We might wonder how problems – especially repeated patterns – can emerge in the face of more and more standards, laws, codes, directives, and policies at the international, federal, and local levels. While some may reflect that the continuation of problems might be due to a need for increased education and training in regulatory requirements, human intuition indicates that something far deeper may be needed. Some of the factors involved in the ongoing problems we see in clinical research may be due to, or at least be aggravated by, a lack of education in areas related to what is commonly referred to as 'values formation'.

While the above reflections clearly indicate a need for educational reform and revision on various levels of instruction, they constitute an even deeper reconsideration of the identity, role, and mission of the CRC/clinical research leader of the future. CRCs regularly, and intensely, interact directly with patients or research volunteers. The CRC is the individual who must often sit down at the proverbial table of research and meet the human volunteer, or touch and analyze data that is connected to living, breathing human beings and their families. Therefore, the CRC is someone who does indeed 'touch the human condition' in ways that are often unavailable, or simply not obvious, to the investigator or medical research and analytical staff.

Since the principles of the "Belmont Report", grounded so clearly in the human condition, are the driving, non-negotiable energy behind human subject protections, it is incumbent on the CRC and other such clinical research leaders to raise the human and humane face of research, and to remind the research industry that its goal is not metrics, but progress ordered towards the good of humankind and not the expanse of human commerce.

Such a role is not merely a job; it is what classical thinkers have referred to as a 'vocation' or a lifestyle choice. This is the stuff of which Nightingale and Schweitzer were made*. It is the stuff of which true healthcare research must be made. It requires the stretching of our self-identity and the caution to be readied for resistance. But can any other pathway be chosen when the opposite choice to human subjects protection looms on the horizon like the dark and sinister silhouette of events that took place at Auschwitz or Tuskegee?

Conclusion

The future direction of the CRC's role must reflect the self-belief of individuals in these roles to remain faithful to their primary mission: to protect humans. CRCs might begin to choose a pathway by addressing the following question: Do we need more laws, or do we need better enforcement and understanding of Good Clinical Practice regulations with a re-emphasis of the principles of respect, beneficence, and justice in trials?

*Florence Nightingale (1820-1920), known as "the lady with the lamp", was a British nurse who was noted for her work during the Crimean war. Albert Schweitzer (1875-1965) was a Franco-German physician and theologian who devoted most of his life after 1913 to a mission in Gabon. He received the Nobel peace prize in 1952 [8].

References

1. Weiss R. About this series. Cosmetic Gene Therapy's Thorny Traits. Science on the Ethical Frontier Series. The Washington Post Sunday, October 12, 1997; Page A01.

2. International Conference on Harmonisation of Technical Requirements for Registration of Pharmaceuticals for Human Use. ICH Harmonised Tripartite Guideline: Guideline for Good Clinical Practice. E6. Available from: www.ich.org. Accessed November 17, 2004.

3. Principles on Conduct of Clinical Trials and Communication of Clinical Trials Results. Washington, DC: PhRMA, 2004:2.

4. National Commission for the Protection of Human Subjects of Biomedical and Behavioral Research. Belmont Report: Ethical principles and guidelines for the protection of human subjects of research. Washington, DC: US Government Printing Office, 1979.

5. Pharmaceutical Industry Profile 2004. Washington, DC: PhRMA, 2004:VII. Available from: www.phrma.org/publications/publications/2004-03-31.937.pdf. Accessed March 21, 2005.

6. Recruiting Human Subjects. Pressures in Industry-Sponsored Clinical Research. Washington, DC: Department of Health and Human Services, Office of Inspector General, 2000:1.

7. Compliance Oversight Branch, Division of Human Subject Protections, Office for Human Research Protections (OHRP). OHRP Compliance Activities: Common Findings and Guidance. Washington, DC: OHRP, 2002.

8. Collins Concise Dictionary, 4th edn. Glasgow: HarperCollins Publishers, 1999.

Standard Operating Procedure (SOP) Template

Standard Operating Procedure *[Title of SOP Topic]*		
SOP number: _____	Category: _____	
Supercedes: N/A – original	Effective date: _____	
Subject: _____		

Written by: _____	_____	_____	
	Signature	Title	dd mm yy
Approved by: _____	_____	_____	
	Signature	Title	dd mm yy
Approved by: _____	_____	_____	
	Signature	Title	dd mm yy

1.0 PURPOSE
[Provide a brief purpose of the SOP.]

2.0 SCOPE
[A general statement of what is covered by the SOP. Include the procedures outlined in the SOP.]

3.0 REFERENCES TO OTHER SOPS
[Cross-reference all SOPs relevant to this SOP.]

4.0 RESPONSIBILITY
[Indicate the clinical research team members who are responsible for the procedures.]

5.0 DEFINITIONS
[Provide a list of terms used in the SOP and include the relevant definitions.]

6.0 PROCEDURES
[Incorporate a short introduction if necessary. Describe the procedures required to implement each activity and divide these into logical categories. Include any documentation requirements.]

6.1. Heading of first activity
[Provide a step-by-step list of procedures. Organize information into easy-to-follow steps.]

6.1.1. Sub-sections [if necessary]
[Include bullet points for additional information relating to a procedure:
- *Essential documents*
- *Adverse events]*

7.0 SOP HISTORY
[In this chart, record the history of the SOP changes. See example below:]

SOP number	Date issued	Summary of revisions
AD-101.001	DD MM YY	Original
AD-101.002		Brief description of revision. Sections of SOP affected.

[Add a brief summary and rationale for the revisions made to the SOP. Include in the chart the SOP effective date, number, and version of the original SOP. Also the effective date and modified version of the revised SOP.]

8.0 APPLICABLE REGULATONS AND GUIDELINES
[List the applicable regulations and guidelines for the SOP, eg, FDA CFR, ICH–GCP, Tri-Council. Include Web sites and links where the information can be found.]

9.0 ATTACHMENTS
[Include attachments as tools that can be used to implement the SOP into clinical research practice. Attachments are usually changed more frequently than the SOP.

- *List associated attachments (ie, forms, checklists).*
- *The attachments are not part of the official SOP document.*
- *Attachments should include a document name and version date in the footer.]*

10. ADDITIONAL BACKGROUND (OPTIONAL)

[*This section is optional and allows the SOP writer to provide additional background information to support the SOP.*]

11. REFERENCES (OPTIONAL)

[*Include a list of relevant published papers. Do not include references to guidelines or regulations as these are already covered in Section 8.0.*]

[*Insert section breaks prior to each attachment*]

ATTACHMENT 1
[*TITLE OF ATTACHMENT*]

[*The headers and footers in the attachments should not be linked to the SOP or to each other, as each attachment will have its own document name and version date in the footer.*]

[*If tables are appropriate, they should be created in Word. Table text may be in Arial font or Arial Narrow, ie:*]

Title		

[*Insert section breaks prior to each attachment*]

ATTACHMENT 2
[*TITLE OF ATTACHMENT*]

Abbreviations

ABPI	Association of the British Pharmaceutical Industry
ACRP	Association of Clinical Research Professionals
ADR	adverse drug reaction
AE	adverse event
CCRC	certified clinical research coordinator
CCRP	certified clinical research professional
CERC	clinical events review committee
CFR	Code of Federal Regulations
CRA	clinical research associate
CRC	clinical research coordinator
CRF	case report form
DCF	data clarification form
DMC	data monitoring committee
EC	European Commission
EDC	electronic data capture
EMEA	European Medicines Evaluation Agency
EWG	expert working group
FDA	Food and Drug Administration
GCP	Good Clinical Practice
HHS	Department of Health and Human Services
HIPAA	Health Insurance Portability and Accountability Act
HRPP	human research protections program
HSP	human subjects protection
ICH	International Conference on Harmonisation
ICH–GCP	International Conference on Harmonisation guidelines for Good Clinical Practice
IEC	independent ethics committee
IRB	institutional review board
NIH	National Institutes of Health

OHRP	Office for Human Research Protections
ORI	Office of Research Integrity
PHI	protected health information
PHS	Public Health Service
PI	principal investigator
PR	public relations
QA	quality assurance
QC	quality control
SAE	serious adverse event
SoCRA	Society of Clinical Research Associates
SOP	standard operating procedure
TSC	trial steering committee

Index

N.B. Pages in **bold** denote material in figures/tables.